TBC30

6 Steps to a Stronger, Healthier You

SECOND EDITION

Michael Wood, CSCS

Foreword by Dr. Hari Khalsa

Wicked Whale
Publishing

The information provided in this book is for general information purposes only. While the author tries to keep the information up to date and correct, there are no representations of warranties, express or implied, about the completeness, accuracy, reliability, suitability or availability with respect to the information, products, services, or related graphics contained in this book for any purpose. Any use of this information is at your own risk. Further, the methods described in this book are the author's personal thoughts and practices. They are not intended to be a definitive set of instructions for wellness, exercise, and lifestyle. Please check with your physician before engaging in any exercise and diet program.

First Edition: November 2017
Second Edition Revised: June 2018

Wood, Michael
TCB30: Six Steps to a Stronger, Healthier You (2nd Ed.) / Michael Wood
Summary: Fitness expert Michael Wood covers an easy-to-follow, six step program on exercise, lifestyle, and wellness for all people to enjoy in this updated and expanded second edition.

ISBN: 978-1-7321925-0-8

Wicked Whale Publishing
P.O. Box 264
Sagamore Beach, MA 02562-9998

www.WickedWhalePublishing.com

Published in the United States of America

PRAISE FOR TBC30

"Michael separates himself from other leading experts in health and fitness through his no-nonsense, easy to understand writing and communication style. This makes applying the information on exercise and nutrition in his book much more likely to stick. This practical and structured approach will support the goal of achieving and maintaining a healthy lifestyle."

Dr. Kyle McInnis
Dean, Merrimack College School of Health Sciences

"Getting fit is kind of like climbing Mount Kilimanjaro, as Michael Wood explains in TBC30. You don't just roll out of bed and do it—instead, you need to set goals, adjust your mindset, and follow a well-designed plan. Wood's wisdom and experience will provide you with the tools and motivation you need to improve your health and fitness."

Alex Hutchinson, PhD, Journalist, @sweatscience, Bestselling Author, *Endure* & *Which Comes First, Cardio or Weights?*

"Working with Michael has been a pleasure. His guidance, support, and knowledge of the fitness industry has been instrumental in helping us grow our business. He gives selflessly, without the expectation of anything in return, the mark of a true fitness professional."

Jacob Rothman, CEO of Perch (www.perch.fit)

"*Michael Wood is simply one of the top trainers and fitness experts in the world, and his enthusiasm is unmatched! In addition to his immense knowledge and experience, he truly cares about his clients, his audience, and his profession. Michael lives his words!*"

J. Henry "Hank" Drought, MS, CSCS*D, NSCA-CPT*D, ACSM EP-C, Owner, USAPersonalTrainers.com

"*The knowledge and techniques used by Mr. Wood are on the cutting edge.*"

Hari Khalsa, DC, Khalsa Chiropractic. On-staff Chiropractic Physician for the Boston Red Sox & New England Patriots.

"*As an integrative medicine physician, looking at the whole person including diet, exercise and lifestyle is part of their prescription for achieving overall wellness. Michael's book, the TBC30 plan, fits the bill in terms of a solid exercise plan and methodology, I would recommend his book and services without hesitation.*"

Erica Song, MD, Owner of Vibrant Life Medicine, Englewood, NJ

"*Michael is able to get inside your head to help you change your body.*"
Sarah Bowen Shea, host of Another Mother Runner Podcast

"We are glad to be featured as an expert in heart rate variability in Michael Wood's new book, TBC30: 6 Steps to a Stronger, Healthier You."

Pavel Pravdin, CEO of the app company Welltory

"His programs are applicable for elite-athletes all the way to the working professional that just want to live a healthy lifestyle. My area of expertise is in the space of performance psychology and Mike has continually displayed an understanding of the connection between the mind and body. He knows that without the mind being in the right place it is almost impossible for the client to truly adopt and succeed with their fitness plan. He takes time in this book, in fact the book leads off with the discussion of mindset, to help the reader better understand the mindset that they bring to exercise. He then follows that with real-life applicable steps to solidify the mindset needed to change habits and behaviors. To make real and lasting healthy lifestyle changes we must connect to them with a healthy mindset - Michael gets this, and so does the TBC30 program!"

Stuart Singer, PsyD, Performance Psychology Coach, WellPerformance, Inc.

"Inspirational and Motivational and best of all ATTAINABLE! Great guide and one I couldn't put down until I read it cover to cover! Smart and well written and a book I will continue to return to."

Amazon Customer (5-Star Review)

Table of Contents

DEDICATION

This book is dedicated to the loving memory of our Angel,

Olivia, who danced her way into Heaven.

You will always be with us.

IIXXVMMIII.

ACKNOWLEDGEMENTS

This book would not have been possible without the help of many people. I'm very fortunate and very thankful to have a wonderful family: my lovely wife Robyn and beautiful daughter Julia, who have had the patience to put up with me during the writing of this book, and the love and support of my parents, Jim & JoAnn and siblings Deanna & David.

To my longtime friend and mentor Dr. Hari Khalsa for writing the foreword for the TBC30 plan.

A special thank you to bestselling, Cape Cod author and publisher (Wicked Whale Publishing), K.R. Conway, who developed the book cover and helped me big time with the second edition of the book. All the great work of Kat Szmit of One Wicked Wordsmith who had the daunting task of editing my manuscript. Thank you to Nathalie Vining and Robyn Wood for their helpful assistance reviewing the author copy of TBC30.

To Rick Kowarek and Erik Phillips from Books by the Sea in Centerville and Vicky Titcomb, owner of Titcomb's bookstore in Sandwich, thank you for all your help with getting TBC30 into your bookstores.

FOREWORD

For over thirty-five years I have been in the healthcare industry, and have seen much change and growth in the types of services offered to patients. Through all the change, an essential profession has emerged: the personal trainer.

As a physician specializing in neuromusculoskeletal conditions, I feel that every patient needs to engage in a dynamic strengthening, stretching and aerobic regime in order to truly obtain their optimal health. Without the proper guidance and supervision, a patient can risk further injury and complication of their condition.

I have had the pleasure of reading Michael Wood's TBC30 Plan. His years of experience, both scholarly and practically, are demonstrated throughout this ambitious text. Michael has many strong attributes that helped him have such a successful company: he has a genuine concern and commitment to his client's physical wellbeing, as well as a keen business savvy that helped him create his loyal customer base. These skills are fundamental in a progressive, growing practice.

I am pleased that Michael is able to share his ideas and years of experience; many can benefit from his thoughtful approach.

Dr. Hari Khalsa
Chiropractic Physician, Khalsa Chiropractic
Cambridge, MA

DISCLAIMER

The information provided within this book is for general informational purposes only. While we try to keep the information up-to-date and correct, there are no representations or warranties, expressed or implied, about the completeness, accuracy, reliability, suitability, or availability with respect to the information, products, services, or related graphics contained in this book for any purpose. Any use of this information is at your own risk. This book is not intended to be a substitute for the medical advice of a licensed physician. The reader should consult with their doctor in any matters relating to his/her health.

INTRODUCTION

"There, ahead, all he could see, as wide as all the world, great, high, and unbelievably white in the sun, was the square top of Kilimanjaro. And then he knew that there was where he was going."

~ Ernest Hemingway, *The Snows Of Kilimanjaro*

T.S Eliot once said, "Only those who will risk going too far can possibly find out how far they can go." I was reminded of those lines when I was getting ready to make a summit push the next morning up Africa's highest mountain, 19,340-foot Mount Kilimanjaro, located in Tanzania.

On the day prior to making our summit attempt I saw a person who had to be carried down the mountain on a stretcher. We found out later that he had been stricken by altitude sickness following a summit attempt. At that

1

moment I remembered thinking *what have I gotten myself into* especially since I had never climbed to high altitude before. I had climbed some smaller mountains around New England over the years but that was about the extent of it. To say that I was a bit worried was an understatement.

My mind began to wander at that moment back to a conversation I had with the owner of Thomson Safaris. This was the adventure travel company based in Watertown, MA, that planned the full itinerary of our wonderful trip.

That particular conversation took place a few months prior to the climb. We spoke about how she thought my body would handle the rigors of high altitude. She told me that she climbed Mt. Kilimanjaro previously with a world-famous climber and film director, David Breashears, who made the film, "Kilimanjaro: To the Roof of Africa."

It sounded from our conversation that he was also a big guy like me and ended up having a bit of an issue regarding the climb. Keep in mind he had successfully climbed Mt. Everest on several occasions (like I had also done...in my dreams). I remember her telling me that I would probably have some issues as well with the altitude due to my size (6'5" 235 pounds at the time). Fortunately, I had no issues and made it up and down the mountain without so much as even a blister.

Our entire entourage lucked out as well especially in regard to the weather the day we made our ascent. The previous day had come with terrible weather and poor visibility. Luckily, our day brought amazing weather with bright sunshine that warmed us, and sadly the glaciers too, during our short stay at the top of Africa's highest peak. I was very fortunate due in large part to the great Sherpa team we had that really took care of us.

The reason I bring up the climb, and the point of the whole story, is to talk about the value of goal setting. Climbing the mountain and reaching the summit was actually a goal that was put in place two years earlier. I wanted to put the goal "out there" to challenge myself.

First, I mentioned it to my wife, Robyn, and some friends while out at dinner one evening. Once it was made public, I knew I would not back down from the challenge or in reaching my goal. A little added pressure never hurt anyone, right?

I gave myself two years to prepare mentally and physically for the climb. Setting short and long-term goals during my two years of training was important in order to build my work capacity and fitness level. I'm not saying you need to go to extremes like I did; there is always value in choosing practical, manageable goals.

Once you have picked a specific, measurable goal, take time to write it down, so you can "own it." This will also help you to follow through. Goal setting can also aide with unexpected outcomes like exercise retention and maintaining motivation during your exercise journey.

In addition to goal setting, adopting the right mindset, completing a fitness assessment, and an overall plan, in my opinion, are all-important and needed for success. Your TBC30 plan will help you with this and more.

I first heard the phrase "commit to get fit" when I started training private clients more than three decades ago. Back then it resonated with me, as it still does today.

An important missing piece in the health and fitness puzzle that was often not addressed in the past, is the commitment to change mindset and behavior.

Another crucial area that is often neglected is fitness testing, or what I refer to as a needs assessment. Management consultant and author Peter Drucker said it best, "how can you manage something if you don't measure it?"

Movement begins between your ears and making a commitment to get in shape requires more than just the physical component; it needs to be in the forefront of your mind. Pick a few reasons that will motivate you to continue your quest to get fit. Write the reasons down and most importantly post them somewhere so you can see them every day.

As an example, one of the top items on my list that keeps me motivated to exercise and stay healthy is my family. I want to be active with them as I age; my goal is to be, as they say, in the game and not watching from the sidelines.

Good luck, believe in the process, and follow the TBC30 game plan that ties in with each of the 6 steps to ensure a successful journey.

CHAPTER 1

Mindset & Assessment

"Eating alone will not keep a man well; he must also take exercise. For food and exercise work together to produce health." ~ Hippocrates

Have you really benefited with the choices you've made when it comes to your diet and exercise? A significant number of people in this country, and worldwide for that matter, who have impaired health and fitness, have certainly not benefited. This is due in large part from an increasingly sedentary lifestyle, coupled with poor nutritional choices (WHO, 2014, and Health Intelligence, 2015). About one-third of adults in the U.S. are physically inactive (Rabin, 2011). The average American spends more than 9 hours a day sitting. Research shows that people who sit the most have a 112 percent increase in the Relative Risk (RR) of getting diabetes and a 147 percent increase in the RR of cardiovascular events compared to people who sit less. Sitting has become the new smoking. It has been shown that sitting for a large part of the day causes similar mortality rates to smoking (Wilmot, 2012). This just adds fuel to the fire adding to the growing list of reasons why more than one-third of U.S. adults are currently obese (35.1 percent or 78.6 million) and 33.9 percent are overweight (JAMA, 2012). When you look at the groups collectively, approximately 70 percent of Americans are either overweight or obese. It's time for a change in mindset, ideally one leading to a different approach, if you're serious about improving the most precious of all commodities: your health and well being.

Let's be honest, we know this can be a very challenging task since most people don't even like to exercise. More than 30 percent of people will not work out at all this year and only 5 percent will exercise at a level that is considered vigorous.

There were about 81.6 million Americans who were completely inactive in 2015. In addition to factors like genetics, emotional instability, and sleeplessness, lack of physical activity is one of the leading causes of obesity. This is one of the reasons why one of the TBC30 goals is to carve out just 20 to 30-minutes most days of the week. That's it! You can find half-an-hour on most days of the week, for the next four weeks, and make a commitment to yourself and your family, right?

> "Given what we know about the health benefits of physical activity, it should be mandatory to get a doctor's permission not to exercise."
>
> **Per-Olof Astrand, MD, PhD, Karolinska Institute, Stockholm, Sweden**

Many government agencies recommend that individuals follow a customized exercise and nutrition plan tailored to their needs and goals to ensure optimal results. It sounds pretty basic but it rarely happens. If you don't set goals, follow a plan, and assess to see if you're improving, the odds are pretty low that you'll continue that journey.

If you're new to exercise or it's been a while since you have exercised on a regular basis then you need to begin slowly. Keep the exercise volume (amount of work) at a low training threshold during the first few weeks of training. The goal and focus during this time period is to develop efficient movement patterns, increase your fitness level and then build work capacity. You will focus on subsequent strength development once those goals are met.

After a specific time period the focus will transition to increasing the volume of training. This is dependent on the needs, goals and chronological training "age" of the person. Any increase in volume or the amount of work (repetitions/sets/load), once again, should not take place until the person has mastered movement competency with each exercise in their current training program.

Movement competency is described as the ability to move free of dysfunction or pain.

The Total Body Conditioning plan (TBC30) is a 30-day diet and exercise plan, based on science, that requires about 30 minutes a day. The TBC30 plan is validated by results. Meaning, hundreds of people before you have tried the plan and as a result have changed the way they look and feel.

One of the goals of the plan is to change mindset and eventually behavior. A key component in regard to changing behavior is "moving from unconscious, automatic reactions to conscious, deliberate decisions."

The program offers a game plan with specific daily and weekly steps that need to be followed in order for this to be triggered and effectively take hold. In addition to moving through the six steps of TBC30, there are also nine diet strategies that need to be followed to improve your chances of success. Making the commitment to exercise regularly and focus on the specific TBC30 diet strategies are important initial steps. The basic concept is to use the plan as a template to bolster commitment and hopefully "ingrain the habits into your brain."

Each step offers a specific game plan to follow over the course of your 30-day plan. Each game plan needs to be incorporated into your lifestyle in order to be successful. <u>The cornerstone of the TBC30 plan is based on the following six principles:</u>

(1) Change your mindset

(2) Perform a needs assessment

(3) Move more

(4) Get stronger

(5) Get leaner

(6) Get more sleep

A by-product of completing your 30-day TBC plan will be an increase in energy level, coupled with improvements in overall health and fitness. You will also find yourself eating more nutritious meals, making better food choices and eating less added sugar.

If this is not the right time for you to begin the program – then hold off – and come back when you can commit the time and energy that are needed for you to be successful.

The TBC30 plan will get you moving down the path that you need to be on in order to get results. This plan, by the way, has worked for hundreds of my private clients through the years, in addition to the many clients who have followed the plan through our online coaching program.

All you need to do is be mindful of the 6 steps that the TBC30 plan is based on. Perform the baseline fitness assessment. Then execute the game plan that is laid out for you over the next four weeks and the plan will work for you too.

Step 1:
Change Your Mindset

"Failure is not fatal, but failure to change might be"

~ John Wooden, former UCLA Basketball Coach

The process of changing a person's mindset begins with determining what type of mindset they actually have. Mindset typically falls into one of two categories, a fixed mindset or a growth mindset.

According to Stanford University psychologist Carol Dweck, PhD, author of the book *Mindset: The New Psychology of Success*, a fixed mindset is where we let failure or even success define who we really are.

Someone with a fixed mindset believes their intelligence and personality are carved in stone and their potential is determined at birth. On the flipside we have a growth mindset, which is someone who ultimately sees setbacks or failures as opportunities to grow and improve. This person believes their intelligence and personality can in fact be developed and their true potential is unknown. According to Dweck, "Cultivating a growth mindset could be the single most important thing you ever do to help you achieve success."

"Your mindset is your collection of thoughts and beliefs that shape your thought habits. And your thought habits affect how you think, what you feel, and what you do. Your mindset impacts how you make sense of the world, and how you make sense of you."

(source: sourcesofinsight.com)

A goal of the TBC30 plan is to bring awareness between the connection of brain, body and breath, referred to as mindfulness. Mindfulness is when you are truly present in the moment, mind and body united.

One activity that has been found to be very helpful in making people more aware of mindset is the practice of yoga. Many yoga classes are meditative or offer a meditation component, typically at the beginning or end of class. This may be a great place for you to start. There are also apps right on your smartphone that can educate you on the psychological and physiological benefits of daily meditation. Two of my personal favorites are *Headspace* and *Calm*.

Many people never reach their health and fitness goals because changing mindset and behavior are not a primary focus.

When a person is not equipped with the right mindset they never reach the point where they are vested in both themselves and the program. The results are goals that never seem to materialize. Sound familiar?

I have stated this time and time again over the course of my career: "It does not matter how good your diet and exercise plans are. If mindset and behavior are not changed, long-terms goals will not be met."

It is important to understand that changing mindset takes time. There is actually an ancient Greek word, metanoia, used to describe such a transformation and it's defined as "the journey of changing one's mind, heart, self, or way of life." You need to first find something that you truly enjoy doing and incorporate that activity into your daily life.

It's not about counting calories, doing a specific workout or following a specific diet. You need to set realistic expectations when it comes to diet and exercise.

Both diet and exercise are seen in a different light when mindset changes. It is now something you're in total control of rather than a chore or something you have no control over. The key is to make it fun and enjoyable.

A 2014 study published in the *Journal of Economic Behavior and Organization* by a group of Australian researchers looked at the relationship between exercise, various personality traits, and other health-related habits.

The researchers found that people who thought they had control over their lives were more likely to exercise and adopt other healthy steps than those who felt that luck or fate largely dictated their lives.

GAME PLAN:

- Determine if you have a fixed or growth mindset.
- Be aware of your entire body during each breath especially during exercise.
- Work on releasing tension in your body while sitting, standing and walking.
- Turn your walking into "walking meditation" and make every step enjoyable!
- Download the Headspace app and find time to meditate for a few minutes each day.
- Download the Welltory app and look at your energy and stress levels using heart rate variability.

SUGGESTED READING:

Dweck, Carol (2016). *Mindset: The new psychology of success*. Ballantine Books: New York.

Harris, Dan (2017). *Meditation for Fidgety Skeptics*. Spiegel & Grau: New York.

Step 2:
Perform a Needs Assessment

"In the end, you won't remember the time you spent working in the office or mowing your lawn. Climb that goddamn mountain." ~ Jack Kerouac

A needs assessment can be defined as the process of identifying and evaluating the needs of a person and possible solutions to problems. It can be viewed as the gap between "what is" and "what should be."

A needs assessment, according to Witkins and colleagues, focuses on the future, or what should be done, rather than on what was done, as is the focus of most program evaluations.

Entrepreneur Peter Drucker has stated often "if you can't measure it, you can't improve it." A good exercise prescription offers a periodic assessment that acts as a check-in and doubles as a motivational tool. This will in turn keep the individual committed and on track with the exercise and diet plan.

I want you to ask yourself what you really want to get out of the TBC30 plan when it's all said and done. Write down your goals, and remember: you don't own them until you actually write them down.

Most people end up starting off on the wrong foot because they do not make, for whatever reasons, any short-term goals when they're program is about to start. Go into your smart phone right now and open up notepad and list your goals or get out your journal and start writing.

A few examples of goal setting could be: to reduce your percent body fat to a specific level, have at least a 2:1 waist-to-height ratio (WHtR), work on lowering your waist-to-hip ratio (WHR) to a specific number, walk a minimum amount of steps each day (like 8,500 steps/day), or climb 10 flights of stairs a day. Maybe your goal will be to limit added sugar, do more push-ups or pull-ups, hold a plank for 2:00 or jog a mile in a specific amount of time.

One of the goals that I personally made this year was to improve my health from the inside out. I'm interested in improving my blood profile or specific biomarkers. Let me ask you - are you the best version of yourself if you are strong and lean on the outside but not healthy inside? For more knowledge in this area I recommend using Insidetracker.com a company based in Cambridge, MA, that I have used since 2013. Use the promo code MWOODFIT for a 10 percent discount when you decide to try Inside Tracker.

Some or maybe all of these suggestions may be the right goals for you to try and improve by the end of your TBC30 plan. That's your call; you know your body best. Again, write it down so you own it. Let's walk through each of the tests that I recommend using in the TBC30 plan and hopefully you decide to use them too. Choose a few of them or all of them, that's your call.

Test 1:

The Waist-to-Hip Ratio

One of the most important areas with regard to your body that needs be measured and monitored is known as your waist-to-hip ratio (WHR). This key health marker informs you if you have unwanted body fat covering your waist and hips.

Researchers refer to individuals who have a high waist measurement as "apple" shaped because weight is typically stored around the abdomen. Individuals who are apple shaped are at a higher health risk than those who carry their weight around their hips (known as "pear" shaped).

Research has shown increases in both waist circumference and WHR, as you age, are associated with an elevated risk of glucose tolerance, diabetes, hypertension, hyperlipidemia and cardiovascular disease.

A study from the USDA Human Nutrition Research Center on Aging at Tufts University suggests that girth measurements are more valid than skinfold caliper readings in the aging population. "Waist and thigh girths, rather than skinfold thicknesses, should be considered for use in longitudinal studies in the elderly because the changes in these girths capture increased abdominal adiposity and sarcopenia, respectively."

The WHR is the circumference of your waist measurement divided by the circumference of your hip measurement (in inches). To obtain the most accurate results I recommend using a Gulick spring-loaded tape measure device.

The waist measurement is taken at the narrowest part of the torso. This is typically below your rib cage and above the hip or about an inch above your navel.

Your second measurement is taken with your feet together, around the widest portion of your hips (see table 1). For example, if you are a male and had a 36-inch waist and 41-inch hips, you would have a ratio of 0.87

and that would place you in the low risk category for heart disease.

Table 1. Waist-to-Hip Ratio (WHR)

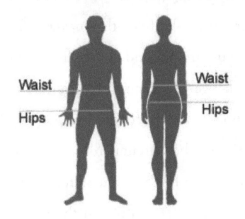

A higher ratio (>1.0) is associated with a greater chance of heart disease. A good goal to have if you are male is less than 0.95 and if you are female, your goal is less than 0.80 for a WHR (refer to table 2). Men should have a waist measurement that does not exceed 40 inches and women should be less than 35 inches.

When your measurement is higher than this, it's usually an indication that you're carrying too much visceral fat that is typically stored deep in the abdominal area.

Research studies have shown that excess visceral fat leads to chronic diseases such as diabetes, cardiovascular disease and metabolic syndrome.

I have always liked and used the WHR because there is a great deal of science-based research that backs up this measurement, and it's pretty easy to do.

I prefer using a Gulick tape measure because it offers a tension-sensing device to ensure reproducible measurements. The Gulick tape measure has been used in sports medicine and anthropometric studies since the early 1980's. This inexpensive device makes it easy for anyone to make accurate measurements as it eliminates the guesswork by applying a known amount of tension (four ounces) to the measuring tape. The Gulick tape measure can be purchased on Amazon for about fifteen dollars.

Table 2. Waist to Hip Ratio Chart

Male	Female	Health Risk Based Solely on WHR
0.95 or below	0.80 or below	Low Risk
0.96 to 1.0	0.81 to 0.85	Moderate Risk
>1.0	>0.85	High Risk

Source: World Health Organization, 1999.

Test 2: Waist-to-Height Ratio

The waist-to-height ratio (WHtR) is another metric, like WHR, that has plenty of strong research behind it that speaks to the validity of the test. The WHtR is basically a distribution of the body fat on your body.

To obtain your ratio simply divide your waist circumference (in inches) into your height (in inches). Make sure you use a Gulick tape measure when you take your waist measurement. For example, a male who has a waist circumference of 34 inches and is six feet tall (72 inches) would have a WHtR of 0.47 which is considered "healthy." Men who score between 0.43 to 0.52, are considered "healthy" and women who score between 0.42 to 0.48 are also considered "healthy."

A study published in 2010 in the *Journal of Clinical Endocrinology & Metabolism* followed 11,000 subjects for eight years before concluding that WHtR was a much better measure of the risk of heart attack, stroke or death than the more commonly used body mass index (BMI).

On a side note, BMI, is not considered the best health marker because it only takes into account your height and weight not muscle mass. Researchers have stated that you should aim to keep your waist measurement less than half that of your height or a 2:1 ratio (both determined in inches).

Test 3:
Track Body Weight (optional)

You may have noticed that up to this point the topic of body weight has not really been mentioned. Obviously, you can monitor your weight if you like – but it's important to understand that it's not just about your body weight. This is because body weight does not offer an accurate snapshot of your body composition and overall health.

The important metrics you should focus on are the amount of muscle mass and body fat you have and what that ratio is. As examples, adult males who maintain 80 percent muscle mass and 20 percent body fat, and adult females who maintain 75 percent muscle mass and 25 percent body fat are considered healthy.

Research from the National Weight Control Registry has shown that members who check their body weight each week are in fact more successful with maintaining a set body weight over many years. But they also do a handful of other things, like walking an hour a day, eating breakfast every morning and watch minimal television.

Try to pay less attention to body weight and focus more on body composition. When body composition is your outcome, the attention shifts to lowering your percent body fat and increasing lean muscle mass.

When you worry less about body weight you begin to notice other things such as having more energy throughout the day or how your clothes all of a sudden fit differently. Maybe you're pulling that belt buckle a little tighter or you went down a dress size. These are much better indicators that are telling you that you're on the right track with your diet and exercise plan.

As you can probably tell, I'm not a big body weight measurement type of guy. Don't get me wrong, I weigh myself, I just understand that there is a standard error of estimation in what the scale reports. We have all had those weekends where our body weight has fluctuated four to eight pounds or more and we know its not because we ate thousands of extra calories. It comes down to your body basically retaining more water.

When you end up having a bad carbohydrate eating and drinking type of night, you know you're going to feel terrible the next morning. When you get up you typically feel bloated around your belly, your face feels swollen, and the skin beneath your eyes is typically "puffy" from water and salt retention. This is usually a result of eating too much processed food, taking in too much salt and lets not talk about drinking too much alcohol.

For every gram of carbohydrate that you consume, the body will store three grams of water.

What you should look at and monitor is the ratio of your current body weight, more specifically, the amount of muscle and fat that you have. Knowing your WHR, WHtR and percent body fat numbers offer a much better picture of health compared to just stepping on a bathroom scale. Don't you think? I know you want to see what your current body weight is, so go ahead and get it done, record it but remember that safe and effective weight loss is no more than one kilogram per week, or 2.2 pounds.

When you lose a great deal of body weight quickly you can bet its not all coming from that extra adipose tissue (fat) that you're carrying. Remember: body weight is not the best indicator of overall health. Knowing your WHR and WHtR and percent body fat offers a better overall picture.

Did you know you could lose about 30-50 percent of your weight from lean muscle mass when you diet and lose a lot of weight over a short period of time? This is why you have always heard that yo-yo dieting is so bad for you and your health, not to mention the negative impact it can have on your metabolism.

Test 4:
Percent Body Fat

There is added value in knowing what your percent body fat is as opposed to your body weight.

The average body fat level for a college-aged male is about 15 percent while a typically female carries about 23 percent and student-athletes can have levels that are half of these measurements.

Essential body fat is approximately 3 percent of body mass for men and 12 percent of body mass for women. The average male baby boomer has a percent body fat level greater than 28 percent while women typically exceed 38 percent.

A realistic goal for men is approximately 13-20 percent body fat and women about 23-30 percent. Your focus should be directed towards how much body fat you're carrying rather than overall body weight. The old pinch test still holds true – if you have an inch or more when you pinch around your waist, for example, you have some work to do.

There are many ways to determine your percent body fat including hydrostatic (underwater) weighing, bioelectrical impedance, DEXA (dual-energy x-ray absorptiometry), and skinfolds. The key is consistency when taking any type of body fat measurement. Make sure the same person does the baseline and follow-up test. You should be able to have this quick test done at your gym or local YMCA.

Test 5:
Record Plank Time

Your first step is to determine what your baseline plank time is. This is basically how long you can hold your body in a plank position using good form. Once you find out your time, you can then work towards increasing your overall "hold" time. This is typically done each week by increasing the time you spend in that prone (plank) position.

Perform the plank three days a week or progress to every other day if you had already been exercising regularly for more than a year. If you have not done a plank before then start on your forearms and if you exercise regularly you may want to try your plank with both arms fully extended. Try to double your initial score by the time you're done with your TBC30 plan.

You know your body best, it's your call, but know that volume typically increases by about ten percent each week when it comes to strength training. You can be slightly more aggressive in terms of building up your (isometric) hold time when it comes to exercises like the plank.

Stuart McGill, PhD, a world-renowned spine biomechanics specialist and a leading authority on core development, says that a two-minute plank is a good goal to shoot for regarding the standard abdominal plank on your elbows.

Record your plank times each week as part of your TBC30 plank challenge. The goal is to challenge yourself three to four days a week depending on your fitness level when starting your program.

Test 6:

Determine a Baseline for Daily Steps

The TBC30 plan recommends using a Fitbit pedometer or a similar product in order to keep track of your daily steps and flight of stairs you climb.

The first step is to find out the total amount of steps that you walk during three consecutive days. Next, find the average steps walked during that time and use that score as your baseline number.

Next, begin adding 500 to 750 steps each week until you reach your personal goal (8,500 to 10,000 is my suggestion).

Finally, work diligently to maintain that level over the course of the four-week program. Also, when possible, try to climb 8-10 flights of stairs each day.

The Harvard Alumni study found that men who average at least eight flights a day enjoy a 33 percent lower mortality rate compared to men who are sedentary.

Your activity level outside of the gym each week is critical. It's not enough to do just a 30-minute workout and then be sedentary the rest of the day; that is what's happening to a lot of people. The idea is to slowly increase your physical activity level using a pedometer or activity tracker (i.e. Fitbit or Apple watch) to help record and monitor. The ultimate goal is to increase your daily movement, above and beyond your exercise session.

There is no significance in terms of trying to walk 10,000 steps each day. The number most frequently seen in publication and studied in exercise research however is 10,000 steps (5 miles). There is an abundance of research showing people who use a pedometer regularly will in fact walk more and are healthier compared to their sedentary counterparts.

A study was completed using a Fitbit pedometer that first hit the market back in 2008. The results showed the average Fitbit user records about 6000 steps a day and according to their website, Fitbit users average 43 percent more steps a day when wearing their Fitbit. The TBC30 plan recommends setting daily, weekly and monthly goals for both total steps and flights of stairs climbed. For example, a typical goal that I like to recommend falls between 8,500 to 10,000 steps a day coupled with a minimum of 10 flights of stairs climbed each day.

A good goal in regard for the number of weekly steps is about 70,000 to 75,000. Keeping track of daily steps can be a great motivational tool and at the same time offer a snapshot of your current activity level, and show whether it needs to be adjusted.

Test 7:

Record & Monitor:

Daily Added Sugar Intake (DASI)

One problem with added sugar is there are no universally accepted guidelines in regard to daily intake for added sugar.

For example, the Institute of Medicine recommends that added sugars make up less than 25 percent of a persons total calorie intake. The World Health Organization recommends less than 10 percent, and the American Heart Association (AHA) recommends limiting added sugars to less than 100 calories a day for women and 150 calories a day for men. The TBC30 plan follows the AHA recommended guidelines but keeps track of grams of added sugar rather than total calories.

Back in the early 1800's Americans consumed about 45 grams of sugar every five days; keep in mind that there are about 35 grams of sugar in one can of soda.

By 2012, that number had grown to 756 grams of sugar every five days, or about 130 pounds of sugar a year if you can believe it.

If you're like most Americans you may be consuming on average more than 600 calories a day from added sugar, equivalent to about 40 teaspoons. More than 50 percent of that comes from soda and fruit drinks. According to Mark Hyman, MD, author of *Ultra-Metabolism*, the average American eats 29 pounds of French fries, 23 pounds of pizza, 24 pounds of ice cream and consumes 53 gallons of soda, 24 pounds of artificial sweeteners, 2,736 pounds of salt, and 90,700 milligrams of caffeine each year.

The Institute of Medicine recommends that added sugars should account for no more than 25 percent of the total calories that you eat, while the USDA has even lower recommendations. They state that the combination of added sugars and solid fats, like butter and margarine, should provide no more than 5 to 15 percent of your daily calories.

One study found a correlation between how high a nation's sugar consumption is and its type 2 diabetes rate. Researchers are now taking it a grim step further by estimating how many deaths can be directly attributed to sugary drinks.

Researchers at Harvard have linked sugary drinks to the deaths of 25,000 Americans every year and 180,000 deaths worldwide. Quanhe Yang, PhD, a researcher at the Centers for Disease Control and Prevention, and his colleagues used national health survey data to examine added sugar consumption as a percentage of daily calories and then determined that there was an association between consumption and cardiovascular disease.

What they found was that as the amount of added sugar in the diet increased, the risk of death from cardiovascular disease also increased. A sugar intake of more than 10 percent to less than 25 percent of total calories was associated with a 30 percent higher risk of cardiovascular death, while an intake of 25 percent or above was associated with a 175 percent higher risk of cardiovascular death.

When you're feeling a sugar craving coming on try to get out for a walk or get in an exercise session. Sugar intake can raise serotonin and dopamine levels, which can factor into your cravings, but exercise can also have a similar effect, so use exercise to combat your sugar cravings!

Your Goal: Consume no more than 2 grams of added sugar for every 100 calories of food that you eat. For men this is approximately 150 calories or 38 grams of added sugar a day while women need only 100 calories or 25 grams a day.

Download the MyFitnessPal app in order to keep track of your added sugar intake each day.

Suggested Reading

Taubes, G (2016). *The Case Against Sugar*. Anchor Books: New York.

Test 8: Heart Rate: Resting/Recovery/HRV

A person's heart beats approximately 4,800 times per hour or 115,000 times over the course of a typical day. You should be aware of three heart rate measurements throughout your training program. They are your resting heart rate, heart rate recovery, and heart rate variability.

The best time to take your resting heart rate in order to get a true reading is before you get out of bed in the morning. Take it over the course of three consecutive mornings and use the average as your baseline resting heart rate. That same heart rate when looked at following exercise can be indicative of a person's fitness level.

Determining heart rate one minute post exercise, specifically, offers great insight into the state of their overall health and fitness. Heart rate recovery following exercise equates to cardiovascular health. The faster your heart rate recovers one minute post exercise the better.

Heart rate variability (HRV) is basically the difference (or variability) between each individual heartbeat. "HRV is commonly used as a global indicator of physiological recovery." A person's HRV score is affected by everything from mindset, to air quality, to age, and even exercise patterns.

This topic has received a great deal of attention lately as seen by the number of articles on the subject that continue to be published in various research journals and media outlets. More importantly, there have been more than 22,000 scientific research papers published on this topic to date.

There is a New York-based company named Welltory that has developed a data-driven app that uses HRV as part of their assessment. According to Welltory, "heart rate variability is a health assessment method based on analyzing the variation in time intervals between heartbeats. It is a non-invasive, objective way to figure out what's happening with your body in real time" (measured in milliseconds, or $1/1000^{th}$ of a second). The app records a resting heart rate taken from your smartphone and then uses its patented algorithm to determine a snapshot of what your energy, stress and HRV levels look like.

You can find out more about the product and company at welltory.com and when you decide to use their subscription service, feel free to use my discount promo code: TBC30. It allows you to get a 20 percent discount on their monthly or annual PRO version of their app.

There are a number of ways you can determine heart rate. A few options include: (1) taking your pulse manually (2) through the use of smartphone apps or (3) wear a heart rate strap. Monitor your heart rate at various points throughout the day and be mindful of how it's affected by exercise, stress, caffeine, or any medication you may be on. Regular aerobic exercise that challenges you over time will help lower resting heart rate. As your heart becomes stronger it becomes more efficient and is able to pump more blood throughout your body but with less effort.

According to exercise scientist Len Kravitz, a University of New Mexico professor, resting heart rate can decrease by 5 to 25 beats per minute with regular aerobic exercise. If you're able to decrease your heart rate from 70 to 60 beats per minute your heart ends up beating 14,400 less times over the course of a day and more than five million less times over the course of a year!

Heart rate recovery is a measurement that looks at how much heart rate falls during the first minute after peak exercise. The healthier a person's heart is the quicker it will return to its normal level; the less healthy the heart is, the longer it takes to recover following exercise.

Monitoring your heart rate is a great way to find out if you're exercising at an optimal level and if so, your cardiovascular system will improve over time. A good way to do this is to keep track of your recovery heart rate following your cardio workout sessions. Record your peak heart rate during exercise and look at how quickly your heart rate recovers following one minute of exercise.

Research shows the faster your recovery the better shape your heart is in. Nishime and colleagues at the Cleveland Clinic found that people with an abnormal heart rate recovery, a decrease of 12 or less beats per minute, were at a greater risk for death from heart disease than those with normal heart rate. According to the study a normal recovery was considered around a decrease of 15 to 25 beats per minute at one-minute post exercise. Other researchers like Watanabe and colleagues have stated as well that heart rate recovery is a powerful and independent predictor of death.

Test 9:
How Strong is Your Grip?

Testing for grip strength is one test that most people may not have tried but there is a reason why many of the longitudinal research studies over the years have used grip strength as part of their testing protocols. Grip strength, measured by a grip dynamometer, is a powerful indicator of over all body strength.

Research has demonstrated high grip strength is associated with a decreased morbidity rate. Low grip strength has been shown by Bohannon to be associated with a greater likelihood of premature mortality. Metter and colleagues have also reported that lower grip strength at baseline as well as declining grip strength over time is associated with increased mortality.

Findings from the 2015 Prospective Urban-Rural Epidemiology (PURE) study looked at and followed nearly 140,000 adults from 17 countries. The study participants had their grip strength measured with a handgrip dynamometer and were then followed for four years. The results, published in the journal *Lancet*, show grip strength is a stronger predictor of death than even systolic blood pressure. The study demonstrated for every 5-kilogram decrease in grip strength there was a 16 percent increase in death overall. They also found a 17 percent increase in both cardiovascular and non-cardiovascular mortality. Finally, as grip strength decreases due to advancing age or inactivity, you can also expect a 7 percent increase in the risk of myocardial infarction and a 9 percent increase in the risk of stroke.

Something that I do that could also help you is to keep a grip-strengthening device in your car. It's great to pull out and use during rides to and from work or especially during any long trip. You can purchase a grip-strengthening device on Amazon and remember what I tell the clients that I coach: if your grip goes...you go, so start "squeezing" and build some grip strength!

Test 10:

Take a Look at Your Ankle Mobility

We lose joint mobility as we age similar to how we lose strength, muscle mass and bone. We know it's inevitable but we can also offset the rate of loss. Regular strength training will offset or retard the loss of strength, muscle and bone. When you do specific mobility exercises on a regular basis you can prevent the loss of mobility that occurs typically in the ankle joint.

There is a quick assessment that you can perform to see how your ankle mobility looks; this is known as ankle dorsiflexion. This movement is important in everyday activities and some of the movements you do at the gym. When a person has limited ankle dorsiflexion they typically have issues with movements like squats, one-legged exercises and landing from a jump.

To test yourself, kneel in front of a wall and bend one knee. The foot that has the knee bent is the test leg. Make sure the tip of the foot on the test leg is five inches away from the wall. You can mark it with tape or use a ruler. From this position, place both hands on the wall and lean in keeping the heel down in contact with the floor. If you can touch your knee to the wall, without lifting the heel, your ankle mobility is OK.

Perform the test on both sides to see if there are differences. If you end up not doing well on the test, it's probably your body trying to tell you to work on mobility more often. Either way, start rolling out the lower leg regularly using a T-Pin Vector or foam roller. You can also use this test as part of your dynamic warm-up routine each time you work out to help increase ankle range of motion and improve mobility.

GAME PLAN:

- Determine your WHR (waist/hip in inches) using a Gulick tape measure.
- Determine your WHtR (waist/height in inches).
- Find your average 3-day step baseline (use a pedometer or watch).
- Plank Challenge – record your baseline plank time.
- Have your body fat taken at the gym using a skinfold caliper.
- Test ankle (dorsiflexion) mobility
- Download the MyFitnessPal app to monitor your added sugar each day.
- Download the Welltory app to monitor energy, stress level and heart rate variability.

The TBC30 plan completed assessment form on page 55 is an example taken from a male client I worked with. The second form, on page 56, is where you'll record your baseline and follow-up test scores.

Test	T1	T2	Delta	Notes
WHR	1.04	1.01	-0.03	Lost 1.5" – goal: <0.95
WHtR	0.52	0.51	-0.01	<0.52
Body Weight	204	196	-8	Goal 185 lbs.
% Body Fat	29	26	-3	Short term goal is 25%
Plank Test	1:30	2:45	+1.15	Great effort!
3-day Step Ave.	7700	9250	+1550	Nice – goal: 10,000 steps/day
Added sugar g/day	105 g/d	56 g/d	-49 g/d	Good work – goal: 38 g/day
RHR	67	59	-8 bpm	Nice!
1:00 post HR	128	118	-10 bpm	Significant improvement
Grip Strength	51 kg	67 kg	+16 kg	Positive score
Ankle Mobility	No touch	Knee touch	passed	Toes are 5" from wall

Additional test options (examples): Blood profile, vertical jump, 1-mile run, 500 meter row, max # pull-ups or chin-ups, etc.

TBC30 Baseline & Follow-Up Assessment Form

Test	Test 1	Test 2	Delta	Notes
WHR				
WHtR				
Body Weight				
% Body Fat				
Plank Test				
3-day Step				
Added Sugar grams/day				
Resting HR				
1:00 post HR				
Grip Strength				
Ankle Mobility				

CHAPTER 2

Movement & Strength

"Physical inactivity is as harmful to your health as high blood pressure, high cholesterol, and smoking."

~ *Steven Blair, PhD*

There is a plethora of published data that backs up the following statement – we are "sitting too much, moving less, and it's killing us earlier than expected."

The TBC30 plan wants to help change this. One way to begin changing it is by bridging the gap between health and technology. The use of technology such as smartphones, activity trackers, and smart clothing, all have the potential to (1) help us move more (2) act as a motivational tool (3) hold us accountable and (4) track, monitor, and award our efforts.

Karyn Hughes, MEd, said it best in a blog post featured on the Cooper Institute website, "tracking, logging, or monitoring devices help us self-correct our behaviors and support consistent behavior change that leads to healthier lives."

Before we discuss the benefits of technology let's first look at what is known as the Hawthorne Effect. The Hawthorne Effect was developed by Henry A. Landsberger and is defined as a change in the performance of a person under observation because they are aware that they are being observed. This is typically why subjects involved in research studies, as well as personal training clients, end up with better results. When a person is cognizant that they are constantly being monitored their chances of success for a specific task improve.

Step 3:
Get Moving

There has been a rapid increase in the use of technology-based activity trackers to promote behavior change and increase physical activity. One of the latest studies, published in 2018, out of the University of California at San Diego, used the Fitbit to follow breast cancer survivors during a 12-week intervention. This is one of the first studies to explore the relationship between the use of a commercially available activity tracker, the Fitbit One, and changes in physical activity.

Fitbit uses a proprietary algorithm to classify each minute of activity as being sedentary, light, moderate, or vigorous activity. The group of 42 women included participants ranging in age from 21 to 85 with an average age of 58 years old. The intervention group significantly increased their physical activity level from baseline, 94 minutes per week, to follow-up, 195 minutes per week over a 12-week period of time.

One of your goals over the next four-weeks is to increase your daily activity level by moving more throughout the day. We know the average person sits about nine hours a day. Your mission, if you choose to accept it, is an easy one – start walking a little bit more each day. Technology is starting to demonstrate through research studies and corporate wellness initiatives that it can help in terms of promoting activity and change behavior. A 2016 analysis revealed that 45 percent of American adults own at least one activity tracker, up from 21 percent in 2014.

You now have a personal goal of 8,500 to 10,000 steps each day (about 5 miles depending on an individual's stride length) or about 70,000 steps a week; a mile is about 2,000 steps. A pedometer can become a great motivational tool that can make and hold you more accountable. You can set a daily or weekly step goal in addition to climbing a specific number of flights of stairs (like 10 flights) and then work hard to try to reach it. I can tell you that there have been many times that I'm so close to my goal that I insist on a short walk with my dog before bed and that, in turn, will push me over the 10,000 step mark for the day.

There is a great deal of evidence that supports the many health benefits of (building up to) 10,000 steps a day. There is a wide range of steps taken by an American adult, which is typically between 2,000 and 12,000 steps per day. The average American takes about 5,900 steps a day while someone whose considered sedentary checks in at less than 2,000 steps a day.

One study showed the average number of steps taken by men was higher in men (7,200 steps/day) compared to women (5,200 steps/day). Individuals who are accumulating more than 12,500 steps per day are considered highly active. A goal of 10,000 steps a day is ideal and the more steps added in with your daily exercise is typically associated with a higher health and fitness level.

One study showed participants who increased their steps to average more than 9,500 a day for 32 weeks lost 5 pounds, 1.9 percent body fat and 1.9 centimeters (0.75 inches) from their hips. They also increased their HDL (good) cholesterol by 3 mg/dl and lowered their body mass index by nearly 2 points. All participants in this particular study increased their steps by an average of 4,000 steps a day.

A research study conducted by Krogh-Madsen and colleagues looked at activity levels using pedometers in healthy, young men. The study found going from 10,000 steps a day down to 1,300 steps a day lowered aerobic capacity by 7 percent and reduced insulin sensitivity by 17 percent compared to a control group in just two weeks.

Stanford University researchers (2007) looked at 26 different studies and summarized the results in the *Journal of the American Medical Association*. Their synopsis showed individuals who use a pedometer take 2,000 additional steps each day compared to nonusers and their overall physical activity levels increase by 27 percent.

A study by Tudor-Locke and Bassett (2004) looked to quantify step activity for a typical day in healthy adults by developing a ranking system. They proposed to breakdown pedometer-determined physical activity into five categories: "(1) <5,000 steps/ day may be used as a 'sedentary lifestyle index'; (2) 5,000–7,499 steps/day is typical of daily activity excluding sports and exercise and might be considered 'low active'; (3) 7,500–9,999 likely includes some volitional activities (and/or elevated occupational activity demands) and might be considered 'somewhat active'; (4) ≥10, 000 steps/day indicates the point that should be used to classify individuals as 'active.' Their final (5) recommendation was for individuals who take >12,500 steps/day and they are to be classified as 'highly active.'

Additional research by Tudor-Locke and Schuna, published in 2012, recommend that adults avoid averaging less than 5,000 steps a day and strive to average greater than 7,500 steps a day, of which about 3,000 steps (representing at least 30 minutes) should be taken at a cadence of 100 steps or more a minute. The added benefit here, according to this team of researchers, it could help prevent type 2 diabetes and treat pre-diabetes.

A sedentary person averages between 1,000 and 3,000 steps a day while the average healthy adult walks about 5,900 steps daily. The average number of daily steps for men was 7,192 and for women 5,210 according to a study published in the journal *Medicine and Science in Sports and Exercise* (2004) by Tudor-Locke and colleagues.

It is not unusual for active individuals to consistently take 10,000 steps a day while highly active individuals can reach 15,000 to 25,000 steps a day and beyond! A pedometer study of an Old Order Amish community showed that their average man recorded 18,000 steps per day while the average woman reached 14,000 steps per day, and it turns out the Amish have one of the lowest rates of overweight and obesity of any community in North America.

The Centers for Disease Control and Prevention (CDC) do not actually say to walk 10,000 steps a day as a goal. The CDC suggests 150 minutes of moderate intensity activity and according to researchers that would equate to about 7,000 to 8,000 steps a day. Having a goal of about three thousand steps above that range would be ideal if weight loss is a goal.

Research published in 2013, in the journal *Lancet*, reported that among people with early signs of pre-diabetes, taking an extra 2,000 steps each day, or the equivalent of a 20-minute moderate-pace walk, helped them lower their chances of heart problems. Over the course of the yearlong study, an additional 8 percent lower risk of heart disease was observed for every 2,000 steps walked a day.

Hippocrates once said, "Walking is a man's best medicine." To find out if his 2,400 year-old remark was actually valid, two scientists from University College London performed a meta-analysis of research published between 1970 and 2007 in peer-reviewed journals. After studying more than 4,000 research papers, they identified 18 studies that met their high standards for quality.

These overall studies evaluated 459,833 test subjects who were absent of cardiovascular disease at the start of the investigation. The subjects were followed for an average of 11.3 years, during which cardiovascular events (i.e. heart attacks and deaths) were recorded. Their meta-analysis makes a strong case for the benefits of good old walking. The group of studies showed that walking reduced the risk of cardiovascular events by 31 percent, and decreased the risk of dying during the time of the study by 32 percent. The benefit of walking was apparent even at short distances (5½ miles per week) and at a slow speed of about 2 mph (an average walking speed is considered 3.1 mph).

Subjects who walked longer distances and walked at faster speeds experienced the greatest protection. Other studies have looked at mood and other health benefits from as little as six minutes of walking outdoors. One such study showed creativity increased by more than 60 percent compared to those test subjects who remained seated indoors.

Suggested Reading:

Neff, G and Nafus D (2016). *Self-Tracking*. MIT Press: Cambridge, MA.

It's Time for a Deeper Look at Your Metabolism

Your body expends calories each and every minute of the day; even when you're sleeping you're burning about 50-80 calories per hour depending on the amount of lean muscle you're carrying.

Metabolic rate, also known as metabolism, is the rate at which your body expends energy. The food that you consume each day comes in the form of carbohydrates, protein and fats. Each of these macronutrients contains a specific amount of calories per gram. A calorie is a unit of energy while energy density is the number of calories in a specific amount of food (see table 1).

TABLE 1: Calorie Breakdown:

Carbohydrate = 4 calories per gram

Protein = 4 calories per gram

Fat = 9 calories per gram

Alcohol = 7 calories per gram

According to Powers and Howley, metabolism is the sum of all the chemical reactions that occur within a living organism, the processes by which compounds are built up or broken down.

Basal and resting metabolic rates (also known as BMR and RMR) are basically an estimate of the amount of calories your body needs to function properly while at rest. It represents the minimum amount of energy (calories) needed for your heart to beat, for your lungs to function properly and to maintain a normal body temperature.

Metabolic rate is typically 6-10 percent lower in women compared to men. Metabolic rate is also affected by age, exercise, stress, temperature, hydration, high altitude, sleep and frequency of meals. Regular exercise, especially strength training, has been shown to slow down the natural decrease of metabolism with age.

The combination of an increase in body fat and the loss of lean muscle can help explain the typical 2 percent decline in a person's BMR per decade throughout their adult years. A longitudinal study by Keys and colleagues also documented a 1-2 percent decline in BMR per decade with age.

There are three requirements needed to obtain an accurate BMR measurement, (1) no food consumed for at least 12 hours prior to testing, (2) no muscular exertion for at least 12 hours and (3) measurement should be taken after subject has been lying down for 30-60 minutes. Roberts and Rosenberg state that "resting energy expenditure is quantitatively similar to the BMR, but it is not subject to all the exacting requirements of a BMR." According to McArdle and colleagues, "basal rates measured in the lab remain only marginally lower than values for resting metabolic rate measured under less strict conditions" (note: most people use the terms basal and resting metabolism interchangeably but they are technically not the same). For our purposes though, we will use the term resting metabolic rate (RMR).

There are three factors that determine how many calories your body needs on a daily basis and the combination is referred to as your total daily energy expenditure (TDEE). These components include RMR, thermic effect of food (TEF) and thermic effect of activity (TEA). Average daily values for TDEE are about 2900 to 3000 calories for men and 2200 for women.

Total Daily Energy Expenditure Formula

$$TDEE = RMR + TEF + TEA$$

The Hidden Benefits of
NEAT and EPOC

The TBC30 plan will focus on two subcategories under TEA, known as, non-exercise activity thermogenesis (NEAT) and excess-post oxygen consumption (EPOC). Most people are not familiar with the terms, NEAT and EPOC.

For our purposes we'll focus primarily on ways that you can increase daily caloric expenditure via RMR, NEAT and EPOC. Your RMR is determined by height, age, gender, and most importantly by the amount of lean muscle that you have. RMR can be reduced with caloric restriction and weight loss in both obese and non-obese individuals.

Women typically have a lower RMR compared to men because they have less muscle mass and a higher percent body fat. An individual's RMR accounts for about 60-75 percent of the total number of calories expended during a typical day and will decrease by about 15 percent when the individual is sleeping.

The body is constantly burning calories while doing everything from breathing to exercise; but did you know it also burns calories when you eat? The additional energy your body requires during the digestive process is known as the thermic effect of food (TEF) and is part of the TDEE puzzle that I mentioned previously making up a small portion of the total calories you need each day. The basic formula for determining your TEF is to multiply the total calories you eat by 10 percent. For example, if you eat 2500 calories a day, you'll burn about 250 calories digesting and processing that food.

Keep in mind though that the effect differs substantially depending on the foods you eat. For example, dietary fat is very easy to process and has very little thermic effect (2-3 percent) compared to protein. The macronutrient, protein, requires your body to work much harder to break down and process the calories resulting in a much larger (30 percent) thermic effect. This is one reason why I suggest that you start to eat more protein with each meal and snack.

One study on the thermic effect of food on lean and obese men showed that RMR and the thermic effect of food at rest, during 30 minutes of exercise, and post exercise, are significantly greater for lean men compared to obese men. The study showed that body composition is a significant determinant of thermogenesis and is basically blunted in obese men when compared to muscular men.

One area where people are able to significantly increase their TDEE is with exercise. Physical activity usually accounts for between 15 percent and 30 percent of TDEE depending on how long and at what intensity you exercise.

As I mentioned previously, the TBC30 plan will focus on two areas that most people are not aware of, NEAT and EPOC. They play a part in the overall plan because of their potential to increase someone's daily expenditure. You have the ability to increase your RMR, NEAT and EPOC. This can be done by strength training, becoming more active throughout the day and increasing the intensity (and duration) of your exercise sessions. The TBC30 plan will train you to do just that.

Percentage of Daily Calories Expended

Resting Metabolic Rate (RMR) = 60-75%

Thermic Effect of Activity (TEA) = 15-30%

Thermic Effect of Food (TEF) = 10%

When exercise intensity and duration are increased the EPOC or "after-burn" will also increase. There appears to be two phases in regard to EPOC. Excess-post oxygen consumption occurs after exercise when the body is returning from elevated levels of expenditure back to normal levels.

The body consumes extra oxygen to help replenish among other things depleted stores of oxygen and glycogen. An exercise session that maintains a higher intensity level and longer duration will require a longer period of time for the body to return back to a pre-exercise or resting level and ultimately more calories will be expended. Though EPOC usually does not typically expend a significant amount of extra calories there are many other acute benefits of chronic exercise, including: decreasing insulin resistance, increasing glucose uptake, and increasing HDL cholesterol levels.

The first EPOC phase includes the first two hours post exercise where the majority of the total calorie burn will occur. The second phase can last from two hours up to 48 or more post exercise, where your metabolism may still be elevated, resulting in additional calorie burn.

Overall, you're talking about just a few hundred calories depending on body weight and the intensity level but it adds up, especially if you're exercising four to five times a week. The more lean muscle a person has, the greater the potential to expend more calories from EPOC.

Non-exercise activity thermogenesis, or NEAT, is the energy your body uses for movement other than exercise. Len Kravitz, PhD defines NEAT as "the energy expenditure of daily activities such as sitting, standing, walking, and talking - all activities that are not considered planned physical activity of a person's daily life." This is an area of research that is starting to get a great deal of attention especially during the past decade. In one research study it was determined that lean subjects (higher NEAT level) expend approximately 350 more calories a day (i.e. walking and standing) when compared to obese subjects (lower NEAT level). That amount of calories over the course of one year would equate to a weight-loss of 36.5 pounds!

When looking at the average person, NEAT accounts for about 30 percent of the physical activity calories spent daily, but for some NEAT can run as low 15 percent in sedentary individuals and as high as 50 percent in highly active individuals.

It is not unusual for someone to sit more than half of his or her waking day and herein lies part of the obesity problem in this and other countries.

A good first step in terms of trying to increase your NEAT is to make a point of standing more at work; especially if you are like most people and have a desk job that requires you to sit in front of computer the majority of the day.

Standing will always burn more calories when compared to sitting (3:1 ratio) and this is one of the reasons why I moved to a standing workstation at the office. A worthwhile short-term goal is to stand an additional hour throughout the day compared to what you're currently doing. As an example, every time you check your emails or make a call, try to do it while standing.

Here is an example of what a typical day looks like for many people but please be sure you don't try to replicate it: The average person drives to work in about a half-an-hour, sits four hours in front of their computer at work, then continues to sit an additional 30-minutes during lunch break, returns to their desk and sits another four hours. After work they get back into their car and drive home but of course it takes longer to get back home due to rush-hour traffic. When they get home they sit down and relax a bit, maybe have a drink, watch the local news and then take a few steps to the dinner table and sit for another 30-minutes. Following dinner they get up and move to the couch and read the newspaper or watch TV for a few more hours and then go to bed and get up again and repeat it all over the next day.

There are many ways to try to offset all this inactivity. Here are a few options you can use to increase your activity level. Stand up for all conference calls. Use the stairs whenever possible. Stand up every half-hour from your computer and walk around the office or take a quick walk around the block. When you know you're going to speak at length to someone then try going out for a "walk while you talk" session. Work on parking your car further away from your location, say yes to walking the dog every night, and my personal favorite, wear a pedometer during the day and set a goal to walk a specific amount of steps each day or over the course of a week.

The cumulative effect of the additional movement throughout your day (via NEAT, EPOC) may be just what the doctor ordered to push you over the "weight-loss hump."

When I mention body composition I'm referring to the different components that make up a person's body weight. The human body is made up of fat-free mass

(FFM) and fat mass (FM), also known as adipose tissue. FFM includes muscle tissue, bone, connective tissue, organ weight, nervous system and fluid.

About 43 percent of total body mass in men is comprised of lean muscle tissue and for women that number is about 36 percent. A pound of muscle is more metabolically active (it requires more calories to maintain) compared to a pound of fat. Muscle also has a higher density level than fat (that is why muscle sinks in water while fat floats) and as a result takes up less space; pound for pound muscle takes up a third less space compared to fat.

When you change your body composition your clothes end up fitting differently and you look "leaner" but you may not see much of a change, in terms of body weight, when you step onto a scale.

You have probably read on various blogs and even in many health and fitness books that building muscle is important (which is true) and that for every pound of muscle you can add you will increase your resting metabolic rate (again, this is true). What is not true, however, is that a pound of muscle burns 50 to 75 calories as reported in books, fitness magazines and blogs in previous years.

We now know that each additional pound of lean muscle tissue actually requires about 6 to 7 calories per pound per day to maintain while a pound of fat requires only 2 calories a day.

I like to think of it this way – a pound of muscle burns three times more calories than a pound of fat, and muscle has greater density. As a result muscle takes up a third less space compared to fat. This is why you look better after months of consistent exercise even if you do not lose much weight (remember: it's not about body weight it's about the ratio of muscle to fat). If your goal is to increase your metabolism you must become more active as you age and build lean muscle with strength training, it's that simple!

It's nice to find out about the bonus we get with NEAT isn't it? There are many positive health changes we can obtain from an increase in NEAT but this can also be erased by inactivity.

A field of study has been developed to look at physical inactivity. It is referred to as inactivity physiology. This is a fast growing field and "the inactivity physiology paradigm says that too little exercise is not the same as too much sitting (physical inactivity) and that too much sitting has very potent effects on the body contributing to many common diseases."

More recently in the Canadian Fitness Survey study, a prospective study looking at mortality over a 12-year period of 7,278 men and 9,735 women (18 to 90 years of age; mean age = 42 years), the authors summarize that there were 759 deaths from cardiovascular disease, 547 deaths from cancer and 526 deaths from other causes (e.g., respiratory diseases, injuries, violence, mental disease, nervous system illnesses and digestive system disorders). After correcting the data for possible cofounders (e.g., adjustments for age, sex, smoking status, alcohol consumption, leisure time and physical activity), the researchers declared that there is a strong association between sitting and mortality risk from all causes, even with physically active individuals. Thus an important finding from this large study is that physical activity does not cancel out the ill effects of too much sitting.

Game Plan:

- Get a minimum of 8,500 to 10,000+ steps a day.
- Complete three 15 to 20-minute interval-based cardio sessions each week.
- Use a heart monitor during all workouts.
- Download the app MapMyWalk in order to help you track your walking. There are also apps if you're a runner, MapMyRun or hiker, MapMyHike.

Step 4: Get Stronger

"Lack of activity destroys the good condition of every human being, while movement and methodical physical exercise save it and preserve it."

~ Plato

The fountain of youth for each of us, in my opinion, can be found in a single word – muscle. You need to build more muscle now because you'll lose it as you age and that loss reduces your strength, balance, functional ability and not to mention your metabolism.

The only way to build and maintain muscle tissue is by strength training on a regular basis. If you do not strength train regularly, as you age, you will become part of the statistical group that loses approximately 5-8 pounds of lean muscle mass with each passing decade starting at about age thirty-five.

The average person can count on three things during their lifetime: taxes, sarcopenia and death. The definition of sarcopenia is the loss of skeletal muscle mass associated with aging.

The term, first coined in 1989 by Dr. Irv Rosenberg at the USDA Human Nutrition Research Center on Aging at Tufts University in Boston, literally means "loss of flesh." To prevent the loss of both muscle and strength (known as dynapenia) as you age, research has shown you must overload your muscles by strength training several times each week to prevent a loss in muscle size and strength.

According to research, individuals who did not strength train lost about 5 to 8 pounds of muscle every ten years, and a by-product of this was a reduction in their metabolism by about 50 calories a day. As you grow older, the loss of muscle mass becomes more pronounced and by the time you reach the age of 70, your muscular system will experienced a 40 percent loss of muscle mass and a 30 percent decrease in strength.

With the loss of muscle mass comes a loss of strength and power. A person's balance, mobility and functionality are also compromised when this loss occurs. Strength appears to peak between the ages of 25 and 35 and is maintained (or decreases slightly) between ages of 40 and 59 and then declines by 12-14 percent per decade after age 50, according to research published by Doherty and colleagues.

During a typical week while on the TBC30 plan you will experience days where you work specifically on strength or get into it with interval-based cardio. You will exercise three days and then take the fourth day off and continue the format throughout the four weeks. Every fourth day should be used as a recovery or active rest day. Try to find time for rolling out, maybe a massage or even myofascial release if necessary. You can purchase a T-Pin Vector or foam roller and use it before or after each exercise session and especially on your recovery days. If you are interested in buying a T-Pin Vector just enter the TBC30 promo code: MWOOD for a 10 percent discount at www.tpinmuscletherapy.com

According to a study published in 1992, women who did not strength train lost about 7 pounds of muscle every ten years and a by-product of this was a reduction in their metabolism by about 50 calories a day. As we age we will continue to lose in the vicinity of 0.5 to 0.8 pounds of lean muscle tissue each year after the age of 40 (or about 8 percent per decade).

Additional research has reported that between the ages of 40 and 50, you can expect to lose more than 8 percent of your muscle mass if strength training is not present.

Research from Nair and colleagues has shown a 3-5 percent loss of muscle mass per decade starting at age 30 for inactive individuals. As you grow older, the loss becomes more pronounced and by the time you reach the age of 70, the muscular system will experience a 40 percent loss of muscle mass and a 30 percent decrease in strength.

This time frame, however, can vary depending on how active you have been. The loss may not sound like much but after a decade you're down five to eight pounds of metabolically active muscle tissue and this negatively effect your resting metabolism as well as your functionality. With the loss of muscle mass comes the loss of strength and power. A person's balance, mobility and functionality are also compromised.

In regard to strength loss, research has shown that there is a 30 percent decrease in strength between the second and seventh decades. Overall, you can expect to lose 50 percent of your current strength level by the time you reach age 80 if you're not strength training consistently.

Research has shown that loss of strength hits the lower extremity (i.e. legs) more severely than your muscles from the waist up. Multiple studies have demonstrated a 20-40 percent age-related loss of leg strength in healthy male and female subjects who were in their seventh and eighth decades of life compared to healthy younger subjects.

The good news is that there is additional research that includes data showing test subjects that added 2 to 6.5 pounds of lean muscle tissue after several months while performing two to three strength training sessions each week.

In a comprehensive research review, Donnelly and colleagues (2003) noted the majority of peer-reviewed resistance training studies (lasting 8 - 52 weeks) have shown increases of 2.2 - 4.5 pounds of lean muscle tissue. This group of researchers suggested that an increase of 4.5 pounds of muscle tissue would probably increase resting metabolic rate by about 50 calories per day. They also thought the most meaningful benefit of strength training during a reduced-calorie diet is that it helps to prevent the loss of lean muscle tissue.

Maybe losing muscle mass does not motivate you enough to exercise more. Hopefully, losing both muscle strength and gaining body fat will do the trick and get the exercise ball rolling.

Researchers have reported a linear increase in percent body fat in men (2.2 percent/decade) and women (3.6 percent/decade) between the ages of 40 and 81 years old. Additional research in this area has demonstrated increases in body fat to be even greater, with men adding 3 percent per decade and women at 5.2 percent increase per decade. This data was reported over an 18-year period and subjects ranged in age from 28-60 years old. Regular exercise and optimum nutrition, however, can help offset these unhealthy changes and it seems we have known this for a very long time.

Back in 1628, William Harvey an English physician stated, "the more muscular and powerful men are, the firmer the flesh; the stronger, thicker, denser, and more fibrous their hearts, the thicker, closer, and stronger are their auricles and arteries."

The bottom line is more muscle equals more strength and improved functionality as you continue to age. More muscle means a higher resting metabolic rate, increased strength and additional calories expended during rest, exercise and everyday activity. Building muscle will also improve your balance and the ability to generate more power and this will decrease your chances of falling as a result of improved functionality.

You often hear how important it is to exercise regularly. The benefits that you hear about are typically received following months of training. Would it motivate you a bit more if you knew that you could obtain significant gains, in both strength and cardiovascular fitness, from just a single bout of exercise?

Well it's true and there is a great deal of scientific literature on the topic. Following an in-depth look at the benefits, I created a list of just a few of the major points that will hopefully excite you the next time you exercise and each session after that!

The next time you don't want to travel to the gym, for whatever reason, think of this list and hopefully it changes your mind. Every workout session does count and is extremely beneficial to your health. Know that there is more behind the scenes and even if there is no change on some bathroom scale, there are plenty of positive changes that are taking place – you just might not see all them right away. The good news is there is a great deal of research showing a single exercise session offers a multitude of protective health benefits.

The Benefits from a Single Bout of Exercise

There has been a great deal of scientific research published showing a plethora of health benefits associated with regular strength training and cardiovascular exercise. Have you ever wondered though if any of those benefits are carried over following a single bout of exercise? The answer is a resounding yes! Here are a few research studies that have looked at this phenomenon.

In a study published in the *Medicine and Science in Sports and Exercise*, researchers found a single bout of exercise—such as 30 minutes of walking—could instantly improve the mood of someone suffering from a major depressive order.

Only 30 minutes of running during the week for three weeks boosted sleep quality, mood, and concentration during the day according to a 2012 study published in the *Journal of Adolescent Health.*

One research study demonstrated just 10-minutes of aerobic exercise improves executive function by priming parts of the brain used to focus on the task at hand, according to this 2018 study published in *Neuropsychologia*.

A review published in the journal *JAMA Cardiology* in 2017 found that between one and three workout sessions per week could provide a "strong" protection for your heart. In addition, one single workout can provide cardioprotection for 2–3 hours up to 24 hours post workout. This cardioprotective effect could be explained by ischemic preconditioning, write the researchers, given that an intense episode of exercise can have systematic effects such as inducing myocardial ischemia.

A study in the journal *PLOS ONE*, showed a workout involving just one-minute of high-intensity activity may not only be beneficial, it may be just as good as a longer moderate-intensity workout.

Researchers from Oregon State University analyzed data on physical activity and other markers of health such as cholesterol and blood pressure for more than 6,000 subjects ages 18 to 85, who had participated in the National Health and Nutrition Examination Surveys (2003-2006). After crunching all the data, the researchers found that 43 percent of people who participated in physical activity lasting 10 minutes or less met federal guidelines for being active. One of the findings showed people who did short bursts of physical activity had an 89 percent chance of not having metabolic syndrome compared to 87 percent of people who met the federal guidelines with structured exercise.

A single bout of moderate intensity aerobic exercise for as less as 30-minutes has been shown it can improve some aspects of cognition, most prominently for memory, reasoning and planning.

In a 2007 study, University of Michigan researchers found that a single cardio workout actually increased the storage of fat in lean muscle mass. This actually improved insulin sensitivity. Low insulin sensitivity, also referred to as insulin resistance, can lead to diabetes if not addressed.

Research shows just one high-intensity interval session (HIIT) per week results in greater cardiovascular gains than multiple moderate-intensity exercise. This is also why two of the three-cardio sessions that you'll do each week with the TBC30 are HIIT sessions. What's more, research suggests that incorporating just one HIIT session per week in addition to a moderate-intensity cardio routine can result in greater cardiovascular fitness gains than moderate-intensity exercise alone.

An acute bout of exercise has been shown to help glucose removal in obese individuals according to a 1990 published paper in the *Journal of Applied Physiology*.

Results published by Swedish researchers following a 2012 study found that among healthy but inactive adults, mere minutes of exercise had the power to alter genetic material in muscle cells.

One study showed that a 20-minute moderate intensity workout had measurable effects on the immune system. Subjects either walked or jogged on a treadmill, depending on their fitness level. They measured levels of TNF, an inflammatory marker, before and after the exercise, and found that there was a 5 percent reduction in the number of immune cells that produced this particular marker.

Well, one thing's for certain – a single bout of exercise can in fact be a pretty powerful thing. The good news is the TBC30 offers twelve strength training sessions on top of that same number of short duration, higher intensity cardio sessions spread over the course of the next four-weeks.

The TBC30 plan will help you increase needed strength and lean muscle, which are lost during inactivity and aging. Always remember the old exercise adage, "use it or lose it," which will always hold true!

Here is what your TBC30 plan weekly schedule looks like for the next four weeks. The idea is to add more movement each week by accumulating more daily steps.

On the exercise front, the idea is to exercise three consecutive days, rest and repeat. This would give you three 30-minute strength sessions, two HIIT and one cardio session each week. Following this format while integrating the nine TBC30 nutritional strategies in a real world setting is ideal. There may be times you fall off the

Day 1	Day 2	Day 3	Off	Day 4	Day 5	Day 6
S	HIIT	S	REST	C	S	HIIT

Note: S = strength day (30:00), HIIT = high-intensity interval training (15:00), C = cardio day (20:00)
The schedule uses a 3-days on and one-day off format that is repeated over a 4-week period. Over the course of a typical week you will perform 3 strength sessions, and 3 short cardio sessions (two HIIT and one interval session).

wagon, life happens, get back on your routine using your 3 days on, rest and repeat routine.

Here is what you can expect from your TBC30 strength training and cardio sessions each week:

Cardio Day: 3x/week, 15-20:00 sessions

During the three days when cardio is required you will perform either traditional steady-state cardio or HIIT.

Two of the three sessions will be HIIT, high-intensity interval training. This type of workout involves short bouts of intense exercise followed by less intense bouts that are repeated for a specific number of rounds.

There is a great deal of research that demonstrates tremendous health benefits of HIIT. This type of short duration, high-intensity exercise is your best bang for the buck. This type of workout can be completed on among other things, a bike, elliptical machine, treadmill, versa-climber, stair-climber, rowing machine, while swimming, running outdoors, on a stand-up paddleboard, jumping rope or sprinting.

According to Kravitz, a researcher at the University of New Mexico in Albuquerque, "HIIT adds up to 15 percent more calories to the total calories expended."

That means if you've worked off 550 calories doing HIIT, you can reasonably expect to burn at least another 83 calories post-exercise.

The TBC30 plan alternates between interval and HIIT sessions. The idea is to rotate between three unique cardio training protocols, all of which are between 15-20-minutes long.

The first session is a 1 to 3 interval protocol. Following a 5:00 minute warm-up, repeat a desired number of intervals using a 1:3 work-to-rest ratio (i.e. 30 seconds of hard effort, followed by 90 seconds at a lower intensity). A typical number of intervals for this type of session are around 4-6 depending on a person's fitness level.

This is followed by an easy cool-down for about 3 minutes. The second option is known as HIIT, high-intensity interval training. This includes a 5:00 minute warm-up followed by a 30-20-10 protocol. This means 30 seconds of moderate work followed by 20 seconds of work using an intermediate intensity followed by 10 seconds of maximum effort for a total of one minute. Repeat this for 8 rounds followed by a 3 minute cool-down. The third option is another HIIT session known as a Tabata protocol. This involves a 5:00 minute warm-up then 20 seconds of an activity using maximum effort followed by 10 seconds of rest. This 2:1 work-to-rest template is repeated 8 times (a total of 4:00 minutes) followed by a 3-minute cool-down.

All three of the workout protocols should take you about 15 to 20 minutes to complete. The exercise intensity will depend on your ability and training history.

The TBC30 plan recommendation is to wear a heart rate monitor during all workouts especially if you're new to exercise. We have this tendency to think we work out hard when in reality the majority of us don't.

Remember the statistic that I mentioned at the beginning of the book: only 5 percent of people who exercise work out at what is considered a vigorous level. Here are descriptions of each of the cardio sessions that you will be cycling through over the course of each week:

TBC30 plan – Cardio Workout Option 1:

1 to 3 Interval Protocol (1:3 work-to-rest ratio)

Cardio Options: Bike, Run, Rowing machine, Versa Climber, ElliptiGO, Jumping Rope, Sprints, Treadmill	
Warm-up = 5:00	Cool-down = 3:00
Choose your equipment, a bike and rower work well. Perform 30 seconds of hard work followed by 90 seconds at a lower intensity. Repeat for 4-6x. Wear a heart rate monitor to see how hard you're working.	
Record Peak Heart Rate	
Record 1:00 post Exercise Heart Rate	
Delta (difference between peak HR & post HR)	

All cardio sessions should be completed on non-strength training days. Complete three cardio sessions each week for the next four-weeks. Two of those sessions will be shorter, more intense HIIT sessions. The third workout, an interval session, should be performed at a lower intensity than the two HIIT sessions. You need to record the following metrics after each session: (1) peak heart rate (2) heart rate one-minute post exercise and (3) the delta between peak and post heart rate. For example, during a cardio session, you recorded a peak heart rate of 165 beats per minute. After one minute, that same heart decreased to 120 beats per minute. The delta, or difference, in this case would be 45 beats per minute.

Over time you want to see this number increase. An indicator of good heart health is when your heart rate can return to 100 beats per minute or less one-minute post exercise. The total time spent on cardio for the entire week should be less than an hour. Remember, more is not better, quality trumps quantity during these three cardio protocols.

TBC30 plan – Cardio Workout Option 2:

30-20-10 Protocol

Cardio Options: Bike, Run, Rowing, Elliptical, Jumping Rope, Sprints, Treadmill, VersaClimber, ElliptiGO

Warm-up = 5:00	Cool-down = 3:00
Perform 30 seconds of moderate intensity work (50%) followed by 20 seconds at higher intensity (75%) followed finally by 10 seconds of maximum effort (100%). This equates to a 1:00 bout of total work. Repeat 8x. Wear a heart rate monitor to see how hard you're actually working.	
Record Peak Heart Rate	
Record 1:00 post Exercise Heart Rate	
Delta (difference between peak HR & post HR)	

TBC30 plan – Cardio Workout Option 3:

Tabata Protocol

Cardio Options: Bike, Run, Rowing, Elliptical, Jumping Rope, Sprints, Treadmill, VersaClimber, ElliptiGO	
Warm-up = 5:00	Cool-down = 3:00
This protocol involves 2:1 work-to-rest ratio. Perform 20 seconds of all-out, maximum effort (100%), followed by 10 seconds of rest. This equates to a 30 second bout. Repeat 8x = 4 minutes total. Wear a heart rate monitor to see how hard you're actually working.	
Record Peak Heart Rate	
Record 1:00 post Exercise Heart Rate	
Delta (difference between peak HR & post HR)	

There are plenty of heart rate formulas to use that can help monitor your heart rate level during exercise. Know that none of them, however, are 100 percent accurate. The scientific research papers where these heart rate formulas were derived from research studies using small sample sizes or were not well designed studies in the first place.

The only way to determine a true maximum heart rate for training would require a stress test. From the results of this type of test you could then determine a pretty accurate heart rate training zone. Once this is determined you would typically exercise at a prescribed heart rate range (i.e. 70-75 percent of the maximal heart rate achieved from your stress test).

You can still use heart rate training zones; just understand they are not accurate. You can also use a Borg Scale that looks at perceived exertion subjectively using a 1-10 or 6-20 scale where one or six are easy and 10 or 20 are maximum effort.

Strength Day: 3x/week, 30:00 sessions

The goal of the TBC30 plan is to develop muscular strength by focusing on primary movements patterns and not specific exercises.

Focusing on just one body part at a time, using specific exercises, would be an effective way to exercise if that was how the human body was designed to move and function. Human movement, however, is not a series of isolated joint actions; the whole body works in concert, for movement to occur.

The TBC30 movements include the Squat, Lunge, Push, Pull, and Carry. Following Phase 1 (weeks 1-4) additional movements, like the Hinge and Rotational movements, may be added to the routine. The key takeaway here is to master the basic movement patterns prior to increasing exercise volume or any type of progression. When the suggested repetition range becomes less challenging (i.e. you're able to do more than 12 repetitions) then increase the weight by about 10 percent.

Build up to 2-3 sets of each exercise using a load that enables you to complete approximately 20-40 total repetitions of each movement by the time you're done with all sets. If you end up working for time instead of repetitions, aim for 30-45 seconds of work per set initially. Perform the exercises in a circuit fashion for about 20-30 minutes.

The goal is to complete the strength sessions three times a week. When an individual has a history of working out, that person has the option of progressing to every other day after the first few weeks.

If you're new to the game, then try 1-2 circuits, 2-3 days a week adding plenty of recovery time between both sets of exercise and the days you exercise. The volume of work that you can complete (i.e., sets, repetitions, load) will depend on your ability and training history.

The TBC30 Exercise Plan
(Phase 1: Weeks 1-4)

The thinking behind the TBC30 plan is that the exercise program is best utilized as a workout template. The goal is to choose specific exercises that meet the needs of the reader. Those particular exercises are then plugged into each of the five movement categories for a given workout session. This is dependent upon what type of equipment you have or may not have. The routine can also be performed using a person's body weight when exercise equipment is unavailable.

Chronological training age is an important item that should be addressed when beginning any exercise program. This is basically the number of years a person has been involved in strength training. Someone who is a novice, for example, would have a chronological training age of zero, which most of the time can be a good thing.

This is because their movement patterns don't have to be "fixed" compared to someone else who has been lifting incorrectly for a number of years. This person has been basically "cementing in or wiring inefficient movement patterns" via their brain and nervous system. That takes time to correct and in most cases is never even addressed. This individual would begin using the lowest recommended training volume when it comes to the number of suggested sets, repetitions or time for a particular exercise set. Someone who has more training experience, or an older chronological training age, may in fact want to be more aggressive at the start and throughout their program. You know your body best. Be smart and train smart.

Dynamic Warm-up:

Each workout session begins by taking time to warm-up the body efficiently prior to starting any exercise session. You should put in additional work on the days when your body experiences any residual stiffness from a prior workout.

The same holds true if you're someone who generally lacks flexibility and mobility. A dynamic warm-up followed by a quick roll on a T-Pin Vector or foam roller can do wonders for your body. Some of the best things to recommend for warm-up are activities like jumping rope, light jogging, back-pedaling, and side stepping. Exercises such as body weight squats, walking hip hikes, walking quad stretch, squat jumps, jumping jacks, mountain climbers, a few push-ups or my favorite, the inchworm (see description), are also recommended.

An Example of a Dynamic Warm-up Build-Up

- Easy Jog (50% effort) for 10-15 yards for all jog/runs.
- Walking Hip Hike – 5-10 yards for all dynamic movements.
- Easy Back Pedal Jog (50% effort)
- Walking Quadricep Stretch
- Run (75% effort)
- Walking Groin Stretch
- Run (75% effort)
- Side-Lateral Step-Over
- Run (100% effort)
- Inchworm

Walking Hip Hike

Stand tall with your pelvis in a neutral position. This occurs when you engage your core by pulling your navel toward your spine while flexing the knees slightly. Next, flex the hip and raise the right knee towards the chest. Grasp the hands underneath the right knee and pull the knee up and in towards the chest. Return the foot to the ground. Repeat on the opposite side. As you perform this action, continue to walk slowly for a specific distance.

Walking Quadricep Stretch

Start by standing with a tall posture with feet shoulder width apart. Flex the right knee bringing the heel towards the buttock. Take hold of your right ankle with your right hand. Pull heel towards the buttock, stretching the quadriceps (front of the thigh). Make sure the right knee does not "wing" out at any time, keep knees close together. Limit any bending at the waist, "stay tall throughout." Raise the left hand overhead for balance.

Repeat on the other side. As you perform this action, continue to walk slowly for a specific distance.

Walking Groin Stretch

Start in a standing posture with feet shoulder width apart. Raise the right leg towards the waist allowing the right knee to drop outward (performing external hip rotation). Take hold of the right ankle with your right hand while the left hand grabs the heel. Now pull the foot upwards towards the waist. Return the foot to the ground. Repeat on the opposite side. As you perform this action, continue to walk slowly for a specific distance.

Side-Lateral Step-Over

Start by standing sideways with knees soft and arms bent and your hands in front of your body. Flex the hip and take the right knee upwards as high as your range of motion will allow. Move the right foot to the right side planting the foot firmly on the ground about a foot from where it was originally. Keep both feet pointed straight ahead throughout the entire drill. Now perform the same action and movement using the left leg. As you're doing this you're moving laterally to the right. Continue to move slowly for a specific distance and then repeat back towards the direction where you began. Visualize stepping over a fence with each step that is about waist height, keeping the foot dorsi-flexed (think "toes towards the nose") throughout the drill.

Inchworm

One of the best full-body movements to perform before a workout is called the inchworm and if I had time to do only one movement before I started my workout, this would be the one.

Start in a plank position with the arms extended and hands directly below the shoulders. Hands should be position about shoulder width and the fingers spread wide and pointing straight ahead. Keep this tight, rigid position throughout (think hard as a board). Keep your core engaged throughout by pulling navel in towards the spine and don't let the low back arch at any time. When you're in the plank position there should always be a straight line running through the ankle, knee, hip, shoulder and ear.

Begin by taking small baby steps while keeping the legs straight. Walk your toes as close to your hands as you can. At this point you're basically in a yoga pose called downward dog. When you're unable to go any further, walk the hands forward a few steps until you're back in the plank position.

Repeat this for a few rounds or about five yards if you're on a marked field or turf. This one movement works your core, ankles, hamstrings, back, shoulders and wrists, basically every muscle group that you are about to use in your upcoming workout. You can also add a push-up or T push-up to the mix as a progression. You also have the option to move in both directions, forward and backward, as you progress.

This type of buildup can be used as a dynamic warm-up template. Obviously, there are a ton of options here depending on what type of facility you're working out at. When you're unable to jog or run because of space issues, simply substitute jumping rope for running. Remember, this is a "warm-up" not a workout so go easy and buildup gradually.

These types of full-body movements will prepare the body for the upcoming workout. This is also where things like balance; flexibility and mobility can be addressed and worked on, sometimes without you even realizing it.

Warm-up & Recovery Tools to Use

There are many different products that can be use to help prepare the body for the demands of exercise.

One such tool is the T-Pin Vector, which is a great muscle therapy tool. Think of it as your mini foam roller - ideal for targeting all those hard to get areas on your body that need to be loosened up a bit. You can also use a traditional foam roller as well. Think about the movement patterns that you're getting ready to work and "roll out" those areas.

These tools are ideal for getting tight muscles to respond better by applying some pressure via the roller and your body weight.

One by-product of all this rolling out is your connective tissues become healthier over time. Connective tissue is made up of your ligaments, tendons and fascia. Fascia is very densely woven and covers every muscle, bone, nerve, artery and vein, as well as, all of your organs including the heart, lungs, brain and spinal cord.

Overtime it can become "sticky" or restrictive from inactivity, too much use, stress, and inadequate hydration to name just a few things.

The goal is to "release" some of the restricted fascia by rolling out the area. There are three types of connective tissue that you should be familiar with:

- Ligaments – connect bone to bone.
- Tendons – connect muscle to bone.
- Fascia – plays an important role in function and support in your body. This support system is actually one continuous structure that covers your entire body, head-to-toe, including all your organs, nerves, bones and muscles.

When rolling-out, remember to move slowly at a rate of about one inch per second. As you roll over especially tight areas simply stop on that area and hold the position for a minute or two. Remember to breathe and try to relax and let go into the position; it can be a bit uncomfortable at times but extremely beneficial.

As the more than 600 muscles in the body begin to move and contract they dissipate heat and the mechanism that is used to cool off the body is called sweating. A good sign that you're ready to exercise is when your body begins to sweat lightly. Think of a dynamic warm-up as the first step needed to turn on your neuromuscular system. As you continue, you will experience a slight increase in heart rate and respiration. This is required to increase the core temperature of your muscles ultimately "warming-up" your body and the synovial fluid in the joints.

As you continue to warm-up, the connective tissue (ligaments, tendons and fascia) also become more pliable. Your movement and agility improve and performance will be better following a dynamic warm-up; it's all about muscle activation.

When you sit all day in front of a computer or do a great deal of driving, muscle will begin to shut off. There is an actual term called "gluteal amnesia" – where the glute muscles actually start to shut off from inactivity.

Sitting all day causes the hip flexor muscles to tighten over time and the glutes to stop firing. This is why you need to spend quality time warming up the body before jumping into a workout after a long day at the office.

Mobility Work

Now that your body is prepared, you can move on to mobility work. Again, there are many things you can do here, the TBC30 plan focuses on specific mobility work that will address areas that are affected by too much sitting, driving and inactivity. The first phase of the plan (weeks 1-4) will focus basically on the back and ankle. Feel free to work other areas of the body that may require your attention. If at any point during the work out you experience any pain beyond normal muscle fatigue, stop.

(1) Kneeling Thoracic Spine Rotation

Begin in a quadruped position. Position knees directly below your hips and place your wrists directly below your shoulders. Hands are about shoulder width in contact with the ground, keeping fingers spread wide. Pull your navel in towards the spine and keep your pelvis in a neutral position. Maintain a neutral position with the head. Move your left hand, placing your hand on the side of the head. Slowly open up rotating your left elbow towards the sky. Exhale as you perform this movement. Push the right hand into the floor as you raise the left elbow towards the sky. The movement should be initiated from the mid-back, the thoracic spine. The thoracic spine sits below your cervical and above your lumbar spine. It consists of twelve individual vertebrae. Perform a desired amount of repetitions and then switch sides.

(2) Side-Lying Thoracic Spine Rotation

Start by lying on your right hip while placing your right forearm on the ground. The upper part of your body (from the waist up) should be off the ground, except your right forearm. Brace your lower body by touching the bottom of your right foot with the left knee. This will prevent you from sliding while performing the movement. Bend the left arm forming a 90-degree angle. Start with the left arm touching the right forearm (which remains in contact with the floor). Next, initiate the movement from the thoracic spine as you move the left arm up over the left shoulder. Your eyes should track your left arms as it moves up and then back to the ground. Keep the involved left arm locked at a right angle throughout the movement, then return to the starting position. Exhale during the exertion phase. Repeat for desired repetitions and then switch sides.

(3) Supine Windmill

Start in a supine position (on your back) with your knees bent, feet flat on the floor and arms spread out away from your body with palms facing up. Pretend there is a piece of rope tied around your legs. Drop your legs to the right until they touch the floor. Next, take your left arm across your body while you rotate your torso.

This is your starting position. It should look like: you lying on your right side, knees bent and on top of each other, both arms extended straight and away from your body. Your arms are at shoulder height and the right palm is facing up while the left palm facing down on top of the right palm (both arms straight). The body is kept (mostly) in that position while you take the left hand off the right and up, across your body until it touches the floor on the opposite side, palm facing up, like the other side. It may or may not touch the floor, depending on the mobility of the mid-back. That is one considered one repetition. Repeat the movement back and forth until you execute the desired amount of repetitions.

(4) Kneeling Ankle Dorsiflexion

This is useful as both a warm-up and test for the ankle joint. As we age we lose mobility in various joints and this is really prevalent in the ankle joint. The ankle joint consists of three bones (tibia, fibula and talus). The foot and ankle contain 26 bones (one-quarter of the bones in the human body are in the feet.), 33 joints, and more than 100 muscles, tendons and ligaments.

Start in a kneeling position about a foot away from a wall. Mark a point that is 5 inches away from that wall. Place the toes of the right foot at the end of that mark (masking tape works well), 5 inches away from the wall.

The left leg should be bent with the knee on the ground. Move the right knee towards the wall. The goal is to move the right knee back and forward until you touch the knee to the wall. The heel of the right foot cannot come off the ground at any time during the test.

A person is considered to have good ankle mobility if they are able to touch their knee to the wall. If not, use this test as a warm-up before you work out and use the T-Pin Vector or foam roller to roll out the back and sides of the lower leg (i.e. the muscles that make up the calf and soleus).

Perform this movement, known as ankle dorsiflexion, for desired repetitions. Switch sides and perform the movement on the opposite ankle.

The goal, when it comes to strength training, is to focus on performing specific categories of movements as opposed to a series of individual exercises. As some coaches like to say, "It's about training movements not muscles."

TBC30 Plank Challenge: 3x/week

At this point you should have a good idea of how long you can "hold" a plank position using good form. The goal, once this is determined, is to work slowly towards increasing your hold time during each workout or increase the overall time at the start of each week for each plank variation.

Start the exercise initially on your forearms, progressing to arms fully extended, if you become less challenged. Try to double your time (from baseline) by the time you're done with your TBC30 plan. You know your body best, it's your call, but know that volume increases typically by about 5 to 10 percent each week when it comes to strength training. The adjustment is usually 5 percent for exercises for the upper body and 10 percent for lower body exercises.

You could probably be slightly more aggressive in terms of building up your hold time when it comes to exercises like the plank. The TBC30 plan recommends a 15-second increase each week. Stuart McGill, PhD, who is a world-renowned spine biomechanics specialist and is considered a leading authority on core development, says that a two-minute plank is a good goal to shoot for regarding the standard abdominal plank on your elbows.

TBC30 plan Core Series:
Bird Dog/Plank/Bridge

Bird Dog

This is a great base level, core strengthening, exercise that has deep roots in the yoga world. Start in a quadruped position. Engage the core by pulling in navel towards spine. Knees are position directly below hips and writs are below shoulders with hands shoulder width and fingers spread wide. Next, extend one leg until it's parallel with the floor and then do the same for the opposite arm. Position the hand so the thumb points upwards. Then perform the same movement with the opposite leg and arm and call that one repetition. Perform the requested number in the 6-12 repetition range depending on the week, building repetitions each week.

Exercise Progression: If and when the bird dog becomes less challenging you have the option of trying to touch the involved elbow to knee. Return to the starting position and repeat.

Prone Plank

Prone refers to the body facing down while supine refers to the body facing up. Start with the feet spread slightly and the arms either (a) extended or (b) bent with the forearms on the ground. In either position, the forearms or hands should be placed directly below the shoulders. The head is in a neutral position with the eyes looking down and slightly beyond your fingertips. Moving from head to toe, maintain distance between the ear and shoulder. Do not hunch your shoulders; focus instead on moving the shoulders away from the ears. Maintain a tight, rigid core by pulling in or bracing your abdominal muscles. Contract the glutes and quadriceps muscles. Maintain a right angle at the ankle joint; keep the toes below the ankle joint, not positioned forward or backward. Maintain a straight line at all times through the ear, shoulder, hip, knee and heel. Hold the position for as long as possible.

Exercise Progression: When either variation of the plank become less challenging you have the option of lifting a foot off the floor for just an inch or two, hold for a desired time or do repetitions and then repeat on the opposite side.

Side Plank

Lie on your left side, with left elbow underneath your shoulder propping you up. The left forearm and hand remain on the floor. Extend your right arm upward or bend the arm and place hand on the hip. Remember to relax your shoulders and don't let your hips drop. Hold for allotted time then change sides.

Exercise Progression: When the side plank becomes less challenging you have the option of raising or abducting the top leg a few inches, holding it for time or repeating for a certain number of repetitions, or just holding the lifted position the whole time.

Glute Bridge

Lie in a supine position (on your back) with your knees bent and feet flat on the floor. You should be able to touch your fingertips to your heels. Before executing the movement, engage your core by pulling your navel in towards your spine; this should flatten out the arch in the lower back. Raise your hips up off the floor until you form a straight-line through the knee, hip and shoulder. Separate the feet slightly. If you have a yoga block or pillow, place it between the knees and squeeze the legs together. Perform for desired repetitions and then slowly lower one vertebrae at a time on the last repetition.

Exercise Progression: When the bridge exercise becomes less challenging you have the option of placing weight on the body (like an Olympic plate or kettlebell) for added resistance or simply straighten one leg so the sole of the foot is facing the ceiling and perform a single-leg glute bridge.

Here is a snapshot of the four core exercises seen in week one that you will complete as part of your exercise routine each time you work out.

Week 1

Exercise	Time	Sets	Reps.
Bird Dog		1-2	6-8
Prone Plank	30 sec.		
Glute Bridge		1-2	8-10
Side Plank	30 sec.		

The bird dog and glute bridge exercises are performed for repetitions while the two plank exercises are held for thirty seconds each. Make sure both right and left sides are completed during the side plank. This has been designed as a circuit format, meaning you should perform each exercise back-to-back without rest, unless you're a novice or deconditioned and may need the rest between sets. The goal during the first week is to perform 1-2 sets of each exercise.

The Five Basic Movement Patterns

The "best" movement options to choose for an exercise program can vary greatly depending on with whom you talk or follow on social media.

The TBC30 plan incorporates five movement patterns in its exercise plan during Phase 1 (weeks 1 through 4). The five categories of movements are: (1) Squat (2) Pull (3) Lunge (4) Push (5) Carry. Specific categories like the Pull and Push have the option of being broken down further into horizontal and vertical components.

For example, 1A. Horizontal Push (i.e. bench press or pushup) and 1B. Vertical Push (i.e. one-arm kettlebell press or push press). The TBC30 plan will do this for the Pull movement category only. This sequence of movements (1-5) that was previously mentioned, is also the actual order used in exercise portion of the TBC30 plan. More advanced movement patterns like the (hip)

Hinge and Rotational movements (or anti-gravity movements) are not included in this phase and can be added at a later point in time (following week 4).

The TBC30 plan does not prescribe specific exercises because the status and past health history of the person reading this book is unknown. Instead, we offer a selection of exercises listed under each block or category of movement.

The first one listed in each category is typically the best exercise to choose during the first few weeks of the program. Exercises mentioned following the first exercise can be used as progressions. Once an exercise can be completed using good form for the desired sets and repetitions, it might be time to progress to a new exercise.

Movement pattern: SQUAT

Squat exercise options: Body Weight Squat, Goblet Squat, Dumbbell Squat, Barbell Front Squat, Barbell Back Squat, Jump Squat, Sumo Squat, or Jump Squats.

Movement pattern: PULL

Pulling exercise options: (combine groups 1A & 1B)

1A. Horizontal Pull: Chest Supported Dumbbell Row, One-Arm Dumbbell Row, Barbell Bent Over Row, TRX Row, Inverted Row, Inverted Row with feet elevated.

1B. Vertical Pull: Lat Pull-down, Assisted Pull-ups (using a band), Chin-ups, Pull-ups, Weighted Pull-ups and Chin-ups.

Movement pattern: PUSH

Pushing exercise options: (choose one each from 1A & 1B)

1A. Horizontal Push: Pushups, Stability Ball Push-ups, Bench Press, Incline Press, T-Pushups, Landmine Shoulder Press.

1B. Vertical Push: Medicine Ball Press, Kneeling One-Arm Press, Military Press, Dumbbell Press, Kettlebell Press, Push Press.

Movement pattern: LUNGE

Lunge exercise options: Split Squat, Reverse Lunge, Forward Lunge, Lateral Lunge, Skater Lunge, Loaded Split Squat, Bulgarian Split Squat.

Movement pattern: CARRY

Carry exercise option: Farmer's Walk (weighted vest), Farmer's Carry (use either Dumbbell, Kettlebells, Olympic plates, Medicine Ball, Sandbag), Unilateral Farmer's Carry, Mixed Grip Carry (hold one dumbbell by side, one overhead), Overhead Carry.

Now that you have a better understanding of the different categories of movement as well exercise options to choose from, here is how it all "flows."

On page 201 you can find the strength templates for week one during Phase 1 (weeks 1-4). The idea is to select one exercise option and plug it into each category for a given week.

Game Plan:

o Increase your activity level (every week). Wear a pedometer and focus on reaching your daily step goal (a minimum of 8,500 to 10,000 + steps a day). Increase daily step totals by 500 to 750 steps each week.

o Strength training/HIIT & Cardio sessions – do both 3 times each week.

o Plank Challenge: Plank 3 times a week.

Chapter 3

Diet & Sleep

"The benefits of exercise are unbelievable...But if you have to exercise to keep your weight down, your diet is wrong."

~ Tim Noakes, MD, University of Cape Town, Africa

STEP 5:

GET LEANER

The majority of people, from my experience, have no idea of the number of calories they're eating. They are also clueless when it comes to added sugar intake over the course of a typical day. With that said, you will need to complete the following two tasks: (1) keep a food journal for 3-5 days, recording everything you eat and drink during that time period and (2) track the number of grams of added sugar you eat on a daily basis.

This is where technology can come to your aide, there are some great apps available that will make your life easier, helping you record and monitor everything from various foods to added sugar. The app that I recommend using is MyFitnessPal. Other helpful apps are: LoseIt, Fooducate and Shopwell.

In order for your body to become lean (i.e. reduce percent body fat) over the course of the next month, you will need to stick to your exercise routine, increase daily activity and follow the nine TBC30 nutritional strategies. Be more cognizant of the quality of food that you're eating as opposed of just mindless eating.

A 2018 study published in *JAMA* found after one-year subjects lost substantial amounts of weight when they focused on food quality, not calories. Both test groups saw improvements in other health markers including waist sizes, body fat, blood sugar and blood pressure levels.

An interesting point to note in this study was how subjects focused on eating specifically whole or "real" foods and they ate as much as they needed to avoid feeling hungry.

The take away from this intriguing study is significant. The findings demonstrated that "people who reduced their added sugar, refined grains and highly processed foods while concentrating on eating plenty of vegetables and whole foods, without counting calories or limiting portion sizes, lost significant amounts of weight over the course of a year."

In order to have a basic idea of the number of calories you currently eat, simply multiply your body weight by the number 14. I'll use myself as an example; 228 lbs. x 14 = 3,192 calories. This is roughly the number of calories I need to consume each day to maintain my body weight. In order to lose weight I would need to create a negative deficit in terms of calories in versus calories expended to lose weight, creating what is known as a catabolic state (break-down).

If I were looking to add a few pounds of lean muscle, I would have to create a surplus in terms of the amount of calories I consume on a daily basis to keep my body in a anabolic state (building). This occurs with consistent, challenging, strength training workouts, quality sleep, a surplus of calories (especially protein) and plenty of recovery between workouts. Losing or gaining body weight occurs through a combination of activity and high quality nutrition. In the past we used the old "500-calorie rule." For example, to lose weight, you were told to expend 500-calories a day through diet and exercise over the course of seven-days, equating to 3500 calories expended and BINGO…you would lose a pound of body weight.

What we forgot along the way was we're not machines, this is not perfect math and all calories are not created equal. When you look at the cumulative effect of calories expended from regular exercise, daily activity (10,000 steps), a high quality diet coupled with caloric decrease, you'll end up being more productive.

A new eye opening study was published this year (2018) in *JAMA* offering new insights on this topic. The study, which lasted a year, looked 600 overweight subjects who met with a nutritionist, exercised regularly and ate a high quality diet. This diet, also called a "foundational diet," consisted of eating more vegetables, whole foods, less added sugar, and less refined grains. The study looked at two groups, one was a low carbohydrate group and the other was a low fat group. Both groups lost on average about 13 pounds and 11.7 pounds respectively. Some subjects lost 50-60 pounds, but that was the average amount lost.

The study determined it's not about counting calories each day or eating a specific macronutrients; it's about the quality of food that you eat on a regular basis. In addition to the weight loss, subjects also experienced improvements in health markers like changes in waist size, body fat, blood sugar and blood pressure – all changing for the better.

A beneficial goal is to focus on becoming more mindful of what you're eating instead of getting into restricted eating or counting calories.

According to Jean Kristeller, PhD, researcher and author of *The Joy of Half a Cookie*, restricted eating can be defined as a "dieting mindset that makes you hyperaware of every morsel you put into your mouth. The restricted eating mindset reduces the enjoyment of eating, socializing, and to some degree, life." Mindful eating is the middle ground between mindless eating and restricted eating. The goal is to find a balance between the two and keep that in the forefront of your mind as you work to incorporate the TBC30 nutritional strategies into the coming days and weeks.

University of California at Berkeley professor and NY Times best-selling nutrition author, Michael Pollan's offers a smart, manageable, diet mantra: "Eat (whole) food. Not too much. Mostly plants."

Speaking of smart and manageable, the following pages show the 9 nutritional TBC30 strategies that need to be followed in addition to regular exercise and moving more throughout your day.

Diet Strategy #1

Drink more water first thing in the morning.

Sufficient water intake has the ability to maintain energy levels, increase metabolism, improve performance and can even prevent feeling hungry. How much water do you really need to drink each day though?

There are a lot of conflicting opinions regarding this question. It seems like we get conflicting reports every time we open a magazine or turn on the news. Various publications continue to present different views on what they think is the ideal amount.

We know that water is the chief chemical component in our body. Our body is comprised of 60 percent water and the majority of that is inside our cells. We eventually need it or we die. We also know that muscle contains about 72 percent water. Many variables come into play when determining how much H_2O our body actually needs on a daily basis, like activity level, health, and environment.

Research has shown that drinking 17 ounces of water first thing in the morning will increase your metabolic rate by about 30 percent over the next few hours. The same researchers believe that individuals who increase their water consumption by just 1.5 liters a day could burn an extra 17,400 calories and experience a five-pound weight loss over the course of a year. In addition to starting your morning off with water, drink a glass or two of water before each meal. This has been shown to not only curb appetite, but in turn you may also end up eating fewer calories over the course of your day. It has been said that "prevention is the best medicine" and this is especially true when it comes to drinking water. It can also be a good idea to substitute water with anything that you may have been previously drinking with your meals. A report from the University of North Carolina at Chapel Hill showed people who drink 7 cups of water a day eat almost 200 fewer calories a day compared to people who drink less than a glass a day.

A review in the journal *Obesity* found that women who were on four very different popular diets lost a greater amount of weight when they drank more water throughout the day.

Water also plays an important role in performance and maintaining balanced hydration levels in the body. Research from the U.S Army dating back to the late 1960's found that being dehydrated by 2 percent caused a 22 percent decrease in time to exhaustion in soldiers. Drinking enough water throughout the day in order to prevent feeling thirsty seems to be sound advice.

Diet Strategy #2
Never skip breakfast.

I want you to start thinking about breakfast as breaking-the-fast ("BreakFast"). Research from the University of Massachusetts Medical School determined that those who skip breakfast are 4 ½ times more likely to be obese compared to people who make time to eat in the morning.

Your breakfast should consist mostly of protein, healthy fats and complex carbohydrate. When you look at the thermic effect of food, it takes more energy (in the form of calories) to metabolize protein compared to carbohydrates or fats.

A 12-week study of overweight and obese women found those who consistently ate a big breakfast, mid-sized lunch and small dinner lost more than twice as much weight as women who took in the same calories, but in reverse order! Those who ate a big breakfast first, also reduced waist circumference, lowered blood glucose, insulin resistance, and levels of ghrelin, the hunger hormone.

Finally, according to a Georgia Centenarian Study, individuals who eat breakfast regularly have lower rates of Type 2 diabetes and are less likely to develop heart failure over the course of their lifetime compared to than those who don't eat breakfast. The study that looked at older Americans over a 13-year period suggests that regularly eating breakfast may lead to a longer-than-average life span.

New research out of Spain has linked skipping breakfast with atherosclerosis or hardening of the arteries. The researchers looked at the breakfast habits and artery health involving 4,000 middle-aged bank workers who at the time did not have heart disease. The researchers found people who skipped breakfast were more likely to have plaque buildup on their arterial walls than those who ate a breakfast containing at least a fifth of their daily calories. This was about 500 calories for a person eating 2,500 calories a day.

Diet Strategy #3
Eat more high quality protein.

Back in the summer of 1988, six years before I began working at the USDA Human Nutrition Research Center on Aging at Tufts University in Boston, I was involved in a groundbreaking research study, not as an exercise physiologist but as a research subject. I was 27 years old at the time and in peak shape. This was also the same year that I worked with my first private client who I was helping come back from a knee injury.

The study, led by prominent researcher Carol Meredith, PhD, was looking at protein metabolism in young men who exercised. There were some pretty big hitters in the field of aging and exercise who worked on this study with her including William Evans, MD and Walter Frontera, MD. A year later their results were published in the prestigious *Journal of Applied Physiology*. The study looked at the effects of exercise on dietary protein requirements. The study included subjects, including yours truly, who were asked to consume 0.6, 0.9, or 1.2 grams/kilogram/day of high-quality protein over three separate 10-day periods while maintaining a constant body weight.

One of the key findings from the study was the data showed that habitual endurance exercise was associated with dietary protein needs greater than the current recommended dietary allowance (RDA) of 0.8 grams/protein/kg/day. This is important because even today this number is still used when informing individuals of daily protein intake. The protein requirement for the two groups of men in the study was 0.94 grams/protein/kg/day. The average age of men in the first group was 26 years old while the second group had an average age of 52 years old.

Research conducted since this study was published has shown both men and women need a higher protein intake compared to what's recommended by most government agencies. In a nutshell, research from protein experts like Stuart Phillips, PhD, have shown the protein requirement should really be more in the area of 1-1.25 grams of protein per kg per day if that individual is involved in regular strength training.

I would ask you at this point – has your diet, especially on the protein side, hurt or helped you in terms of building lean muscle mass? If you have been involved in strength training and eating like a champ but have not seen a change in the way your body looks and feels, you're most likely not taking in enough protein. Don't feel bad; a lot of other people are in the same boat with you.

What should you do? Start by becoming more aware of what you're eating on a regular basis. Start by building each meal around a lean protein, making sure you are eating plenty of whole foods, vegetables, some fruit, healthy grains and fats.

A nice goal to start with is to consume about 25 grams of protein per meal. Make sure to drink plenty of water too. Try eating smaller meals every 3-4 hours and if you still have issues look into taking a protein powder, like Ascent Protein, a clean, native whey, post workout. Another option, try a slower releasing casein powder prior to bedtime.

Diet Strategy #4
Don't drink your calories.

Consume the majority of your calories from food not beverages such as soda, sports drinks, and alcohol. It has been reported that the average American drinks more than 60 gallons of soft drinks each year. The average person in the U.S. consumes 450 to 550 calories a day through drinking beverages like fruit juices, sports drinks, soda and alcohol. It was determined in 2006 that 21 percent of the calories that Americans consumed came from soda, juice, milk, beer, or other beverages and that that number was up from 16 percent since the 1970's. According to the Beverage Guidance Panel, published in a 2006 issue of the *American Journal of Clinical Nutrition*, a healthy diet should rely on food, not fluids, to provide an individual's daily calories and nutrition.

This may help explain the results of a study by a group of researchers from Harvard University and Children's Hospital in Boston. The study was conducted across eight years involving nearly 50,000 women. The researchers found that women who increased their intake of sugar-sweetened beverages, like soda or fruit punch, from one per week to one or more per day increased their caloric intake by a whopping 358 calories a day and gained a significant amount of weight. The group of women who reduced their intake cut 319 calories per day and gained less weight. Previous studies demonstrated that consumption of sugar-sweetened soft drinks increased the likelihood of obesity in children but this is the first long-term observational study in adults that showed the same findings seen previously in children.

Diet Strategy #5
Be aware of processed foods.

You know the deal here, "if it's white don't bite," be aware of items such as white bread, white rice, etc. White food generally refers to foods that are white in color and have been processed and refined, like flour, rice, pasta, crackers, cereal, cookies and simple sugars like table sugar and high fructose corn syrup. Many of these processed foods are made of saturated fats and large amounts of sodium and sugar. The natural, unprocessed white foods, like egg whites, cauliflower, turnips, onions, white beans are not included in this category.

I have had the pleasure of hearing Walter Willett, MD, speak on several occasions regarding different nutritional topics while working at Tufts Research Center on Aging in Boston. "Fat is not the problem," says Dr. Walter Willett, chairman of the department of nutrition at the Harvard School of Public Health. "If Americans could eliminate sugary beverages, potatoes, white bread, pasta, white rice and sugary snacks, we would wipe out almost all the problems we have with weight and diabetes and other metabolic diseases."

Research from Harvard University published in the *New England Journal of Medicine* followed subjects over a 20-year period and determined that the food most often associated with weight gain was...you guessed it, white potatoes.

Again, don't focus on restricted eating; just be more mindful of what you're eating throughout your day. Make note of how you feel and how your body is reacting when you eat certain foods.

Diet Strategy #6
Decrease your added sugar and salt intake.

The average American consumes about 40 teaspoons of sugar each day (about 600 calories) and this far exceeds what your body needs. The American Heart Association recommends the amount be cut to a maximum of six teaspoons (100 calories or 25 grams) a day for women and nine teaspoons (150 calories or 38 grams) for men. According to Robert Lustig, MD, author of *Fat Chance*, and a leading expert in childhood obesity at the University of California, San Francisco, School of Medicine "sugar is not just an empty calorie, its effect on us is much more insidious. It's a poison by itself."

Dr. Lustig and colleagues have also shown, through their research, that for each additional 150 calories of added sugar consumed per day, above daily requirements, was associated with a 1.1 percent increase risk of type 2 diabetes. A 2013 review of 68 different studies found "consistent evidence that increasing or decreasing intake of dietary sugars from current levels of intake is associated with corresponding changes in body weight in adults" (*BMJ*, 2013). When you really want to lose weight, exercise and cutting your added sugar intake is a great place to start.

Start reading food labels and become more aware of the sugar content in everything you eat. There are a few great apps that you can use to help you monitor your added sugar intake like MyFitnessPal, Fooducate, Sugar Rush and LoseIt. Watch out especially for sucrose (table sugar), fructose (sugars found in fruits), and high fructose corn syrup (HFCS), a mixture of glucose and fructose, and can be found in everything from ketchup to Gatorade.

One study that was completed at the University of California at Davis, found adults who consumed 25 percent of their daily calories from HFCS for two weeks had increase levels of cholesterol and triglycerides, indicators of increased risk for heart disease. In 2011, researchers at Georgia Health Sciences University concluded that high fructose consumption by teenagers could potentially put them at risk for heart disease and diabetes.

The outlook doesn't get much better when we shift our attention to daily salt intake. It may be hard to believe but the average person consumes more than 6000 milligrams (mg) of salt each day. That is about 2.5 times the recommended amount of 2400 mg a day. According to the American Heart Association, individuals should "reduce their sodium intake to 1,500 mg per day and not exceed 2,300 mg per day." But most of us get 1.5 teaspoons (or 8,500 mg) of salt daily. This translates to about 3,400 mg of daily sodium. It is true that your body needs a certain amount of sodium, but too much can increase blood pressure and increase the risk of heart disease and stroke.

Eating more than 2,300 mg of salt per day could raise your blood pressure to unhealthy levels. If you're someone who already has high blood pressure, your doctor may recommend that you keep your sodium intake below 1,500 mg a day. Finally, remember that your body only needs about 3.8 grams of salt per day so don't be like most people and consume 7 to 8 grams a day.

Diet Strategy #7
Be aware of portion distortion.

Watch your portion size during each meal and for any snack; this is an easy way to consume extra calories over the course of a day. If you are eating out at a restaurant and the size of the meal is too big, take a quarter of the meal home in a doggy bag and you will eliminate 500 calories or more. Think about portion sizes as the size of your fist or for the sports fans out there, the size of a hockey puck, for each food group you have on your plate.

Speaking of plates, start to use smaller plates, bowls and glasses when you eat. Bigger portion size and "super-size" can be found at most fast food chains – so for the next four weeks work hard to eliminate any fast food you typically eat.

One lunchtime meal at McDonald's can wreck your day, not to mention your waistline, with one of their 1600-calorie meals.

Diet Strategy #8
Eat more fruits and vegetables.

We know intuitively that we should eat more fruits and vegetables. We have heard it our whole lives. Now you need to simply follow through and do it. Many fruits and vegetables are considered super foods and are rich in antioxidants, high in fiber, vitamins, minerals, and low in calories. The key word here is fiber and by increasing your daily fruit and vegetable intake you'll improve your chances of consuming 35-38 grams/fiber/day for men or about 25-28 grams/fiber/day if you're a women. Another way to look at this is to eat 14 grams of fiber for every 1,000 calories that you consume.

Many nutritionists recommend at least five to nine servings of fruits and vegetables a day. The problem is that Americans get less than five servings a day. Focus on getting a little more fiber (and protein) in your meals and snacks and you'll find yourself less hungry between meals.

Diet Strategy #9
Decrease your calories prior to bedtime.

If all else fails, make sure you at least follow this last strategy over the next four weeks (in addition to of course cutting back on added sugar). Your goal is to avoid any "empty" or non-nutritional calories 3-4 hours prior to going to sleep. This especially includes foods or drinks that contain any caffeine or alcohol.

This may be difficult for some of you because of busy work schedules or because you need to entertain clients for work and they typically eat and drink later in the evening. You might find that the quality of your sleep will improve if you cut out caffeine, alcohol and any extra calories after dinner. Many of us seem to do well during the day when it comes to caloric intake; it usually ends up being late night when those extra calories seem to sneak in there. Even a few hundred extra calories each night, collectively over the course of a week, could be the culprit for weight gain.

The TBC30 Top 22
Super Foods & Drinks

There is an abundance of healthy food and drink options that are available to you. The following alphabetical list includes some of the most often cited products found in nutrition books and scientific research papers. The TBC30 plan recommends eating these healthy foods, fruits, vegetables and drinks.

Avocado – Research has shown they can help prevent unwanted inflammation. One cup of avocado provides about 7-8 grams of dietary fiber. It is the only fruit that provides a substantial amount of what are known as MUFA's – healthy monounsaturated fatty acids. Avocados are a naturally nutrient-dense food that contain nearly 20 vitamins and minerals like vitamin A and potassium.

Apple – Are loaded with vitamins and fiber. The average fiber intake in the U.S. is only 17 grams a day for men and 13 grams for women and it should twice as much as those numbers, eating more fruit, like an apple, will help. The phytonutrients and antioxidants that are contained in apples may help reduce the risk of developing cancer, hypertension, diabetes, and heart disease.

Asparagus - Is rich in fiber and also contains a considerable amount of protein (4-5 grams/cup). This veggie is packed with healthy vitamins and minerals, such as vitamins A, C, E, K, and B6, as well as folate, iron, copper, calcium, and fiber. Four asparagus spears contain 22 percent of your recommended daily allowance of folic acid. Asparagus contains high levels of the amino acid asparagine, which can act as a natural diuretic. Eating more asparagus spears can help flush excess fluid and salt from your body, which can help to prevent urinary tract infections. A 2009 study published in the *Journal of Food Science* suggested that the minerals and amino acids found in asparagus extract may help ease any hangover and protect your liver cells from toxins found in alcohol.

Beet – Beets are a good source of fiber, which is beneficial for digestive health, as well as reducing the risk of a number of chronic health conditions. I have always been intrigued for some reason with the health benefits of beets. Studies have shown that beets can significantly lower blood pressure by up to 4–10 mmHg over a period of only a few hours after eating them. Beets contain a high concentration of nitrates, which have been known to lower blood pressure. This may help in terms of reducing the risk of heart attacks, heart failure and stroke. Several studies have also suggested that dietary nitrates may enhance athletic performance; this is probably why I really like them. In two studies in men, 17 ounces (500 ml) of beet juice daily for six days extended time to exhaustion during high-intensity exercise by 15–25 percent, which equates to a 1–2 percent improvement in overall performance. Eating beets may enhance athletic performance by improving oxygen use and time to exhaustion. To maximize their effects try eating beets or drinking beet juice 2 to 3 hours prior to training or competing.

Berries – Are loaded with antioxidants, especially Blueberries. The berries that give you the most antioxidant bang for the buck are, in order: cranberries, blueberries, blackberries, and raspberries. A 2013 study found that women were less likely to have a heart attack over an 18-year period if they ate more than three servings of strawberries or blueberries per week.

Cauliflower – Is high in folate - A recent study in the *British Journal of Nutrition* found that foods that are high in folate help individuals lose 8.5 times more weight when dieting. A 2007 study published by the National Academy of Sciences found that sulforaphane could protect a person's skin from ultraviolet radiation damage. Cauliflower has a high sulforaphane content and this helps fight against skin cancer, inflammation, and cell damage.

Brussel Sprouts – One of my favorites. One and a half cups of brussel sprouts contain about 430 milligrams of omega-3 fatty acids. Brussels sprouts come packed with Vitamin C, E, A and dietary fiber, each 1-cup serving offers about 4 grams of fiber. One cup of brussel sprouts contain the following:

o   56 calories

o   4 grams protein

o   4 grams fiber

o   274 percent vitamin K

o   162 percent vitamin C

o   24 percent vitamin A

o   24 percent folate

o   18 percent manganese

o   14 percent potassium

o   14 percent vitamin B6

o   12 percent thiamine vitamin B1

o   10 percent iron

o   270 mg of omega-3 fatty acids

Cruciferous Vegetables - like Kale - Broccoli - Broccoli Rabe – All three are loaded with vitamins, minerals and rich with antioxidants. These vegetables are also rich in potassium. Researchers at the USDA Human Nutrition Research Center on Aging, at Tufts University, found that foods rich in potassium help preserve lean muscle mass. In another study published by South Dakota State University's Department of Health and Nutritional Sciences in 2014 discovered that a naturally occurring chemical called phenethyl isothiocyanate (PEITC), found in cruciferous veggies may prevent a relapse of certain cancers such as cervical cancer.

Eggs – You always have one item on a list like this that is controversial. Eggs have gotten a bad wrap for a long time. You should eat the yolk...wait, no you should not eat the yolk. One large egg contains 6 grams of protein and 9 essential amino acids. The World Health Organization ranks eggs at 100 percent for "high biological value" because of their incredible amino acid content. They are one of the few food sources on the planet that contain vitamin D. Eggs are also rich in iron, phosphorous, selenium and vitamins A, B12, B2 and B5, to name a few. One complete egg does contain 185 mg of cholesterol and the recommended daily allowance is 300 mg for healthy adults. To be safe, you may want to eat just one egg if you have high cholesterol and then go with egg whites. One thing doctors and nutritionist do seem to agree on though is it's definitely worth spending the extra money or time to find pastured eggs, ideally purchased directly from a farm when possible. Stick with organic, cage-free eggs for the highest nutritional content.

Figs – Are a good source of potassium, a mineral that helps to control blood pressure. There are also 5 grams of fiber in three servings. One dried fig gives you 3 percent of your daily calcium requirement and 2 percent of your daily iron. The American Diabetes Association recommends figs as a high-fiber food that helps promote functional control of diabetes.

Fish – Eat fish at least twice a week, especially wild-caught Alaskan Salmon (do not eat farmed Salmon) and Mackerel. Sardines offer 21 grams of protein (3 oz.) plus an abundance of other nutrients. Freshwater trout is recommended by the American Heart Association and is high in omega-3s and low in mercury. Avoid certain fish like Tilapia, Bluefin tuna, Mahi Mahi, Grouper and Marlin due to a variety of factors, including high levels of mercury, excessive PCBs, and general overharvesting by fishermen. Bluefin tuna, for example, has the highest levels of mercury compared to any other tuna and is severely over harvested according to a report found in the *New York Times*. A better tuna option would be albacore tuna, which has a lower mercury level.

Research has been shown eating fish regularly can help ward off prostate cancer, depression, and poor eyesight. These particular types of fish should be avoided because they either contain high levels of mercury, they are loaded with PCB's or are being over harvested by fishermen. Bluefin tuna for example has the highest levels of mercury compared to any other tuna not to mention it's severely over harvested according to a report found in the *New York Times*. A better tuna option would be albacore tuna that has a lower mercury level.

Grapefruit - Is an excellent source of vitamin C, a vitamin that helps to support your immune system. Grapefruit is low in calories and provides a significant amount of fiber, vitamins, minerals and antioxidants. Grapefruit juice is ranked among the highest in antioxidant value and it helps reduce insulin levels in your body. That is pretty powerful. A 2006 study in the Journal of Medicinal Food, involving 91 obese subjects, found that those who consumed half of a fresh grapefruit prior to meals lost significantly more weight (3.5 pounds over 12 weeks) than those who didn't eat grapefruit.

Green Tea - Men who drank the most green tea were found to have an 86 percent reduced risk of prostate cancer compared to those drinking the least amount. Research suggests that drinking 5 cups a day can increase your body's metabolism and help you lose more weight around the abdominal area.

Mushrooms - Mushrooms have been found to be very effective in preventing breast and prostate cancer due to the presence of beta-glucans and conjugated linoleic acid. Japanese researchers found that Shiitake mushrooms can lower blood cholesterol up to 45 percent. There are approximately 140,000 different species of mushroom-forming fungi in the world, but science is only familiar with about 10 percent of that number. Research has shown that there are many health benefits to eating mushrooms, such as lowering cholesterol, improve bone health, boosting immune system, lower blood pressure, increase iron absorption, and mushrooms help on the diabetes front, to name a few. My favorites are Portobello and Shiitake mushrooms.

Nuts – Researchers from Georgia Southern University found that eating a high-protein, high-fat snack, such as almonds, increases your calorie burn for up to 3 and a half hours post consumption. Research on people who ate pistachios for 3 months lost 10 to 12 pounds on average. A study from Harvard University's School of Public

Health showed that people who ate nuts had a lower risk of coronary heart disease than those who rarely or never ate nuts. Some of the best types of nuts to eat are almonds, walnuts and pistachios. Just watch the amount that you eat – a handful will do – they are very calorie-dense.

Quinoa – (pronounced KEEN-wah) – Quinoa is an amino acid-rich "complete protein" seed. It is also a good source of riboflavin, which is necessary for energy production within cells. The seeds offer good amounts of protein, fiber, and various vitamins and minerals, including high levels of magnesium, iron, B-vitamins, calcium, potassium, phosphorus, vitamin E, and various antioxidants. Quinoa is also gluten free and often recommended for those on a gluten-free diet. There are 100 different types of quinoa. A 1955 study published in the *Journal of Agricultural Food Chemistry*, titled "Nutritive Values of Crops, Nutrient Content and Protein Quality of Quinoa" substantiated the various nutritional powers of quinoa.

Red Wine – Red wine is loaded with antioxidants, particularly flavonoids like quercetin and resveratrol. Red wine is the only alcoholic beverage included as part of one of the best diets in the world, the Mediterranean Diet. Women should consume one 8 ounces glass per day and no more than two 8 oz. glasses a day for men. One 5 ounces glass of red wine has 0.81 grams of sugar.

Spinach – This amazing green, leafy vegetable is high in niacin and zinc, as well as protein, fiber, vitamins A, C, E and K, thiamin, vitamin B6, folate, calcium, iron, magnesium, phosphorus, potassium, copper, and manganese. Factor Co-Q10, which is an antioxidant present in spinach, plays a key role in strengthening muscles, especially the heart muscle. According to the *Journal of Cardiovascular Nursing*, Co-Q10 can be used to help prevent and treat various cardiovascular diseases such as hyperlipidemia, heart failure, hypertension and coronary heart disease.

Steel-cut Oats – Avoid cold cereal because of its high added sugar content and substitute with a hot bowl of oats. This will give you energy and keep you fueled up all morning long. Add a few walnuts, a banana, blueberries and sprinkle on some cinnamon (great for stabilizing blood sugar levels) and some almond or coconut milk. Oatmeal is filled with stress-fighting and immune-boosting zinc. Stay away from oatmeal that comes in a box or a package – it has too much added sugar. Steel-cut oats may take a bit longer to cook but its well worth it. A serving of oats are considered a "power food" because they are an excellent source of protein (5-6 grams). They also contain, soluble and insoluble fiber (8 grams) not to mention B-vitamins, and calcium while low in sodium and unsaturated fat. Finally, one of the most significant health benefits of steel-cut oats is that they help eliminate fat and cholesterol from your body. Research shows that individuals with high cholesterol (above 220) who consume just 3 grams of soluble oat fiber per day can lower total cholesterol by 8 to 23 percent. This is significant because each 1 percent drop in cholesterol translates to a 2 percent decrease in the risk of developing heart disease. The benefits of steel cut oats exceed the benefits of rolled oats because of the way they are processed.

Sweet Potato - Sweet potatoes are high in many important nutrients including vitamin A, vitamin C, Manganese, vitamin B6, and Potassium, to mention a few. One large sweet potato contains more than 100 percent of the daily recommended intake for vitamin A, according to the U.S. Food and Drug Administration. They are also a great source of B6 vitamins, which help break down homocysteine, a substance that has been shown to contribute to hardening of blood vessels and arteries, according to Harvard University School of Public Health. Eating sweet potatoes have also been reported to (1) stabilize blood sugar levels, (2) promote vision health, (3) boost brain function, (4) can help with weight loss, (5) bolster immune system and (6) are high in antioxidants. I'll have some of that.

Tempeh – Is a soy-based protein that is packed with fiber and other nutrients. Tempeh is low in sodium and a serving of tempeh contains more fiber than most people consume in one day. It can help reduce cholesterol in the body and contains manganese that helps on the diabetes front. A scientific review published in *The American Journal of Clinical Nutrition* evaluated 11 studies that were conducted over a 16-year period. The researchers found that soy isoflavones, which are found in tempeh, significantly decreased serum total cholesterol and LDL cholesterol levels.

Tomatoes – Have an impressive amount of vitamin A, vitamin C, and vitamin K, as well as significant amounts of thiamine, folate and vitamin B6. They are also a good source of potassium, manganese, magnesium, copper and phosphorus. Lycopene, one of four plant compounds found in tomatoes, is a red pigment and antioxidant, which has been extensively studied for its beneficial health effects. One group of researchers have found a connection between the antioxidants found in lycopene and bone health.

Tomatoes are usually red when they are mature, but can come in a variety of colors, including orange, yellow, purple, and green.

Bonus - **Dark Chocolate** – Has many reported health benefits coupled with a high antioxidant content. Cleveland Clinic research has found that flavanols have a positive effect on heart health by helping lower blood pressure and improving blood flow to the heart. Flavanols are the main type of flavonoid that is found in dark chocolate. The key is eating dark chocolate that contains at least 70 percent cocao. Before you get too excited though, if you're the type of person, like me, who at times, has trouble eating just one small piece – then don't buy it and keep it in the house. The average American consumes about 12 pounds of chocolate a year.

Game Plan:

o   Follow the 9-Nutritional Strategies.

o   Focus on reducing added sugar. A goal for women is <100 calories (25 grams) of added sugar a day. A goal for men is <150 calories (38 grams) of added sugar a day.

o   Increase the amount of daily fiber. You can use the same numbers, in terms of grams, that you used for added sugar as a goal when monitoring your fiber intake. This could be 150 calories (38g) and 100 calories (28g) respectively for men and women.

Step 6:
Get More Sleep

"It is a common experience that a problem difficult at night is resolved in the morning after the committee of sleep has worked on it."

~ John Steinbeck

Did you know if you live to 75 years old, you end up sleeping away 25 of those years or 9,125 days? The sixth and final step requires you to get more uninterrupted sleep. It is one of the most important steps in the program because proper "recovery" is critical. When your body is given plenty of time to recover, through adequate sleep, it runs optimally. Sleep is essential to willpower and willpower always comes in handy when you're trying to be more mindful of diet and exercise through good decision making.

We have become a sleep-deprived society and the evidence supports this, showing that we sleep on an average 6.8 hours as opposed to 9 hours a century ago. About 30 percent of adults report sleeping less than 6 hours per night.

A study published in the *Canadian Medical Association Journal* showed that individuals who got less than 5.5 hours of sleep each night lost 60 percent more lean muscle that those who got adequate sleep. Another study from the University of Colorado showed subjects that got minimal sleep on consecutive nights gained two pounds on average over the course of the study.

A second study from the University of Pennsylvania Sleep and Chronobiology Laboratory looked at the sleeping and eating behavior of 225 people. They reported in the journal Sleep, when you're awake between the hours of 10 p.m. and 4 a.m., you're more likely to consume extra calories. The group ate an average of 553 more calories, typically choosing foods higher in fat, when they were kept awake until the early morning hours.

The most valuable assets you have are your body and mind and both require a certain amount of sleep each night to function optimally, yet 60 percent of the population is not sleeping well throughout the night. Start to think of sleep as a time to restore your body and mind. This is critical because without a sufficient amount of sleep each night, your body will not be able to perform at an optimal level.

Research has shown that people who get less than six hours of sleep a night have higher blood levels of inflammatory proteins than those who get more than six hours. This is important because inflammation is linked to diabetes, stroke, heart disease, arthritis, and premature aging, according to a data published in the Centers for Disease and Control and Morbidity and Mortality Report.

Research conducted in 2004 has shown that sleep deprivation can enhance the release of specific peptides in the body that produce hunger. Men that slept only four hours each night for two days witnessed a decrease in specific hormones such as leptin and an increase in ghrelin compared with men who slept ten hours during that same time period. Leptin is an appetite suppressant hormone that is produced by adipose (fat) tissue, and ghrelin is released from the stomach in response to someone fasting and promotes the feeling of hunger. The hormone leptin acts on the central nervous system, most notably the hypothalamus, by not only suppressing food intake but stimulating energy expenditure as well. Ghrelin levels typically increase before meals and decrease after meals. This particular hormone stimulates appetite as well fat production and can lead to increased food intake and a gain in body weight.

A growing number of researchers are beginning to think the obesity epidemic in this country may be caused partly by lack of sleep and the effect this has on specific hormones. In addition, if you're going to bed late, the odds are you're up watching late night television with Jimmy Fallon or Jimmy Kimmel and involved in mindless snacking. There is nothing worse than a few late night calories before going to bed. Additional research from the University of Chicago and the University of Wisconsin has shown that subjects who monitored their caloric intake and averaged 5.5 hours of sleep had more body fat compared to subjects who were consistently getting 8.5 hours of sleep. The National Sleep Foundation's sleep recommendations of 7-9 hours of uninterrupted sleep for adults (ages 18-64) and 7-8 hours of sleep for older adults (age 65+) were updated in 2015 and published in *Sleep Health: The Official Journal of the National Sleep Foundation.*

Finally, the Wisconsin Sleep Cohort Study looked at more than 1,000 subjects and found those who slept less than 8 hours a night had an increase in BMI that was proportional to decreased sleep. This group of researchers also found that shorter sleep times were associated with an increase in circulating ghrelin and decrease in leptin, a pattern that is consistent with low energy levels.

Are you wondering right about now what a good definition of sleep might be? Glad you were wondering because according to William Dement, MD, author of *The Promise of Sleep*, there are two essential features that distinguish sleep from various sleep-like states. The first is that it occurs naturally (i.e. no sleeping pills) and the second is that it is a daily occurrence in humans. When you're not getting adequate amounts of sleep you're likely to go into sleep debt which according to Dement is the accumulated loss of sleep over a length of time. It is like a monetary debt and it must eventually be paid back.

One final comment on the importance of sleep and it is explained nicely in the book, *Biological Rhythms and Exercise*: "Weight-training exercises may be unaffected by partial sleep loss early on in a training session, but the performance suffers due to lack of drive and concentration as the (exercise) session continues."

As you begin to add the six steps from the TBC30 plan into your daily routine, you will start to notice your energy level is better throughout the day and while exercising. The final step, Get More Sleep, is one area that many feel like they can neglect but as I previously mentioned it's probably one of the most important steps, especially since the other five steps are so dependent on this step, so, you may want to start focusing on this critical step starting tonight.

A good Sleep Self Assessment Quiz can be found on the following website:

www.talkaboutsleep.com/sleep-self-assessment-quiz/

Game Plan:

o   Eliminate all products containing caffeine (coffee, chocolate etc.) by mid-day to ensure a good sleep.

o   Sleep goal for adults: 7-9 hours of uninterrupted sleep (18-65 year old).

o   Sleep goal for older adults: 7-8 hours.

o   Perform a Follow-up Assessment.

o   Download the Sleep Cycle app to help monitor your sleep and offer some insight on how you're sleeping.

Suggested Reading

Dement, W. (2000). *The Promise of Sleep*. Dell Publishing: New York.

WEEKLY EXERCISE PLANS

TBC30

For video clips of all the following exercises, please go to MichaelWoodFitness.com or scan the QR code below with your smart phone..

Exercise Descriptions for Weeks 1-2

Movement Category: SQUAT

Exercise: Med Ball Squat.

Maintain a tall standing posture with feet shoulder width apart and feet turned slightly outward. Hold the medicine ball at chest height touching the body. Relax your shoulders and position your elbows downward towards the floor. Maintain a strong core. Sit back and then flex your knees until your thighs are parallel to the floor. Pause for a second then extend the hips and knees returning back to the starting position. Push your feet "through the floor" during the return phase of the movement. Push your knees outward during the return phase as well.

Movement Category: SQUAT
Exercise: Goblet Squat.

Hold a kettlebell at chest height. Elbows should be pointing downward towards the floor. Position your feet about shoulder width apart. Maintain a strong core. Start by sitting back as though you were attempting to sit in a chair. Do not let the kettlebell come off the sternum area. Then flex the hips and knees and lower towards the floor. Touch your elbows to the top of your thighs. Pause for second and return to the starting position. Push your feet "through the floor" during the return phase of the movement. Push your knees outward during the return phase as well.

Movement Category: PULL

Exercise: Chest Supported Row.

You have the option of supporting your chest and upper body on an incline bench or, if you don't have a bench, then perform a bent-over row. In this position, keep your core engaged, knees bent, and arms extended down by your sides holding a dumbbell in each hand. From either position, the exercise is basically the same. Bend your arms and pull from your elbows. Pull both elbows to the ceiling, pause for a second, and return slowly to the starting position. Repeat for the desired amount of repetitions. Again, if you have no bench available then perform a bent-over row using both arms. This is essentially an unsupported bi-lateral row.

Movement Category: LUNGE
Exercise: BW Split Squat.

This is a great exercise to start with in the Lunge series because you're not moving your body forward/backward or side-to-side as with other lunge exercises. Position your feet shoulder width apart before moving your left foot slightly back and the right foot about three feet in front of you. Maintain a tall posture. Bend both knees while moving the body downward. Lower the body until the left knee touches the floor or the right thigh is parallel with the floor. After a slight pause, begin to move the body back up to the starting position. Focus on pushing the front heel into the ground on the way back up. Make sure the front knee does not override the toes.

Movement Category: Horizontal PUSH
Exercise: Push-ups.

This is considered a great staple exercise and should be done prior to attempting any exercises using a dumbbell or barbell. You should be able to handle your body weight prior to moving towards weights. Position yourself the same way as though you were getting ready to hold a plank. The goal is to maintain a straight line through the ear, shoulder, hip, knee and ankle. Eyes should be looking down, slightly beyond your fingers. Position the hands slightly wider than the shoulders. Try to keep your elbows in toward your body. To help you with this, try to "corkscrew" your hands into the floor (i.e. rotate them clockwise a few degrees) before you begin. Then slowly lower the body towards the floor. Pause and return. Move at the speed of a slow controlled breath. Inhale during the lowering phase and exhale during exertion or the extension phase.

There are different schools of thought for foot positioning. Try keeping the feet together and the buttock contracted throughout the movement.

Movement Category: CARRY

Exercise: Loaded Carry.

You may not be as familiar with this category of movement but it's a good one because it works your core, improves grip strength, hits a lot of different muscle groups and even builds work capacity. There are a lot of ways you can go here in terms of what you can carry and how you carry it. Meaning, you can use dumbbells, kettlebells, Olympic plates, a sandbag etc. and these items can be held down by your side, overhead, one by your side and one overhead etc. Stand tall with a tight, rigid posture holding weight in each hand with your arms down by your side. Keep knees soft, core engaged, and shoulders down and retracted (squeezed together). That part is very important. Walk in a straight line for a desired time. Keep head up and eyes straight ahead, do not look down. Do not use a heavy weight at first. Work on getting your form and technique right.

Movement Category: Vertical PUSH
Exercise: Dumbbell Alternating Press.

This exercise can be done standing, sitting or kneeling on one knee. Try standing first. Start in a tall posture, knees soft, core engaged and a dumbbell in each hand. Flex your arms, like you're doing a Hammer Curl, and position the dumbbells at shoulder height, palms facing each other. Extend the right elbow pushing the weight upward. At the top of the movement your arm should be back not forward. The right bicep should be back near your ear. Slowly return the weight to the starting position and repeat on the opposite side. That is one repetition. Complete the desired amount of repetitions. Keep the weight light initially until you have mastered the movement.

Exercise Descriptions for Week 3-4

Movement Category: SQUAT

Exercise: Barbell Back Squat.

Position an Olympic bar (choose either a 22.5-lb. or 45-lb. bar) across your upper back and take hold with both hands. Feet are positioned at shoulder width with the feet turned outward jut a few degrees. Maintain a raised chest and retracted shoulder blades as you lower the weight until your thighs are parallel to the floor. Then drive the feet into the floor and extend the knees and hips as you return back to the starting position. Remember to corkscrew your feet into the ground and drive your knees outward during the ascent. If you do not have a barbell you can use dumbbells.

Movement Category: PULL
Exercise: One-Arm Dumbbell Row.

There are two options for performing this exercise. In option A you will bend your left leg and place it on a bench while the right leg is straight with the foot on the ground and knee slightly bent. Support yourself by keeping your left hand on the bench as well. Hold a dumbbell in your right hand with the arm extended downward. Maintain a straight back and core engaged. This is your starting position. In option B the setup is the same as above except both feet are on the ground and knees are kept slightly bent. Your left arm is still supporting your body weight. The right arm is holding the dumbbell. Next, retract or squeeze the shoulder blades together, then focus on pulling the elbow towards the ceiling. Continue to pull the dumbbell up in towards the outside of the right chest and shoulder. Pause for a few seconds, focus on contracting the back muscles and then slowly lower the dumbbell back to the starting position.

Movement Category: LUNGE

Exercise: Reverse Lunge.

This exercise is a great multi-joint exercise, meaning you're working multiple muscle groups around different joints, in this case the knee and hip.

Start in a tall position, feet hip-width apart and hands on your hips or out in front of you. Keep the left foot where it is. Take a big step backward with the right foot. Then bend both knees simultaneously, lowering the body down towards the floor. Build up until you're able to get the front right thigh parallel to the floor. Push off the ground and return the right foot next to the left foot. Repeat the same movement on the opposite side. One repetition is completed after a movement is completed on each side.

Movement Category: Horizontal PUSH
Exercise: Bench Press.

Lie in a supine position (on your back) on a bench with your feet flat on the ground. Take hold of the bar with a slightly wider than shoulder width overhand grip. Lower the bar to the mid-chest area and then drive the bar upward back to the starting position. It's important to maintain four points of contact during the exercise: keep the head, shoulders, buttock and feet in contact with the bench and ground. Perform the movement at a slow, controlled speed, matching your breath with the speed of the bar. Inhale on the way down and exhale on the exertion phase as you push the bar upward.

Movement Category: Vertical PUSH
Exercise: Push Press.

Stand tall, core engaged, and dumbbells in front of the shoulders with palms facing each other. Next, bend the knees in order to drop the hips (hip flexion) before quickly extending the hips to help drive the weight overhead. Return the weight back by the shoulders and repeat. This exercise can be performed with dumbbells, kettlebells or a barbell.

Phase 1: Week 1 – Strength Session Template

Exercise	Time	Sets	Reps.
Squat		1-2	6-8
Pull		1-2	8-10
Lunge		1-2	6-8
Horizontal Push		1-2	8-10
Carry	30-seconds		
Vertical Push		1-2	8-10

The chart above shows the various movement patterns. The chart on the next page has an exercise listed under each movement category; take note that there is a subcategory listed under the Push offering a horizontal and vertical component that needs a selection for both. This is also typically seen in the Pull category but the TBC30 combined both in that particular block.

TBC30 Plan - example of a week 1 workout session

Exercise	Time	Sets	Reps.
SQUAT: Goblet Squat		1-2	5-8
PULL: One-Arm DB Row		1-2	8
LUNGE: Split Squat		1-2	6-8
Horizontal PUSH: Bench Press		1-2	8
Loaded CARRY: Farmer's Walk	30-seconds		
Vertical PUSH: DB Alternating Press		1-2	8

The first series of exercises seen below is an example of what a workout would look like after you choose the appropriate exercises for your body and plug them into the appropriate movement block:

o SQUAT: Goblet Squat.

o Horizontal PULL: One-Arm Dumbbell Row.

o LUNGE variation: Split Squat (using body weight).

o Horizontal PUSH: Bench Press.

o Loaded CARRY: Farmer's Carry (using either a kettlebell, dumbbells, or weight plates).

o Vertical PUSH: Dumbbell Alternating Military Press.

Week 1: Repeat each for 1-2 sets (for desired repetitions or time).

TBC30 Plan: Phase 1: Week 1 Template

Exercise	Time	Sets	Reps
Warm-up			
Dynamic Warm-Up			
T-Pin or Foam Roller	5:00		
Mobility & Core			
Mobility work (4)	5:00		
Bird Dog		1-2	6-8
Prone Plank	30-sec.	1-2	
Glute Bridge		1-2	8-10
Side Plank	30-sec.	1-2	
Movement			
Squat option		1-2	10-12
Pull option		1-2	8-12
Lunge variation		1-2	8-12
Horizontal Push option		1-2	8-12
Weighted Carry	30-sec.	1-2	
Vertical Push option		1-2	8-10

TBC30 Plan: Phase 1: Week 2 Template

Exercise	Time	Sets	Reps
Warm-up			
Dynamic Warm-Up			
T-Pin or Foam Roller	5:00		
Mobility & Core			
Mobility work (4)	5:00		
Bird Dog		1-2	6-8
Prone Plank	45-sec.	1-2	
Glute Bridge		1-2	10-12
Side Plank	45-sec.	1-2	
Movement			
Squat option		2	10-12
Pull option		2	10-12
Lunge variation		2	10-12
Horizontal Push option		2	10-12
Weighted Carry	45-sec.	2	
Vertical Push option		2	8-10

TBC30 Plan: Phase 1: Week 3 Template

Exercise	Time	Sets	Reps
Warm-up			
Dynamic Warm-Up			
T-Pin or Foam Roller	5:00		
Mobility & Core			
Mobility work (4)	5:00		
Bird Dog		2	8-10
Prone Plank	60-sec.	2	
Glute Bridge		1-2	12-15
Side Plank	60-sec.	1-2	
Movement			
Squat option		2-3	10
Pull option		2-3	8-12
Lunge variation		2-3	8-10
Horizontal Push option		2-3	8-12
Weighted Carry	60-sec.	2-3	
Vertical Push option		2-3	8-12

TBC30 Plan: Phase 1: Week 4 Template

Exercise	Time	Sets	Reps
Warm-up			
Dynamic Warm-Up			
T-Pin or Foam Roller	5:00		
Mobility & Core			
Mobility work (4)	5:00		
Bird Dog		2	10-12
Prone Plank	75-sec.	2	
Glute Bridge		1-2	12-15
Side Plank	75-sec.	1-2	
Movement			
Squat option		3	8
Pull option		3	8
Lunge variation		3	8
Horizontal Push option		3	8
Weighted Carry	75-sec.	3	
Vertical Push option		3	8

Week 1/Day 1

Choose a weight for each exercise that will enable you to complete the suggested repetition range for each exercise listed in each movement category. Each exercise should be performed at a slow, controlled pace. Eliminate any momentum during the execution of all exercises. If you're a novice exerciser try using your body weight as your resistance. As an example, you could use your body weight for Squats, Split Squats and Push-Ups for the respective Squat, Lunge and Horizontal Push movement categories. When you're able to perform more than the suggested number of repetitions, increase the resistance by no more than 10 percent.

Week 1/Day 2

Repeat the same workout flow that you did on Day 1. If an exercise was too easy add resistance or if you used body weight, perform the movement at a slower cadence to keep your muscle under tension longer. This is known as TUT – time under tension.

Week 1/Day 3

Repeat the same workout as the previous two days. If you were doing one set of each exercise, progress to two sets.

Coaching tip: for best results wear a heart monitor.

Nutrition tip: for best nutritional results consume a whey protein drink, like Ascent Protein powder within 30-90 minutes post exercise. Or if you make a shake, add the protein (25 grams) and a banana or another fruit to the mix to get some carbohydrates as well.

TBC30 Plan: Phase 1: Week 1 / Day 1

Exercise	Time	Sets	Reps
Warm-up			
Dynamic Warm-Up			
T-Pin or Foam Roller	5:00		
Mobility & Core			
Mobility work (4)	5:00		
Bird Dog		1-2	6-8
Prone Plank	30-sec.	1-2	
Glute Bridge		1-2	8-10
Side Plank	30-sec.	1-2	
Movement			
Med Ball or Goblet Squat		1-2	10-12
Chest Supported Row		1-2	8-12
Body Weight Split Squat		1-2	8-10
Push-ups		1-2	8-12
Loaded Carry	30-sec.	1-2	
Alternating Press		1-2	8-10

TBC30 Plan: Phase 1: Week 1 / Day 2

Exercise	Time	Sets	Reps
Warm-up			
Dynamic Warm-Up			
T-Pin or Foam Roller	5:00		
Mobility & Core			
Mobility work (4)	5:00		
Bird Dog		1-2	6-8
Prone Plank	30-sec.	1-2	
Glute Bridge		1-2	8-10
Side Plank	30-sec.	1-2	
Movement			
Med Ball or Goblet Squat		1-2	10-12
Chest Supported Row		1-2	8-10
Body Weight Split Squat		1-2	8-10
Push-ups		1-2	8-10
Loaded Carry	30-sec.	1-2	
Alternating Press		1-2	8-10

TBC30 Plan: Phase 1: Week 1 / Day 3

Exercise	Time	Sets	Reps
Warm-up			
Dynamic Warm-Up			
T-Pin or Foam Roller	5:00		
Mobility & Core			
Mobility work (4)	5:00		
Bird Dog		1-2	6-8
Prone Plank	30-sec.	1-2	
Glute Bridge		1-2	8-10
Side Plank	30-sec.	1-2	
Movement			
Med Ball or Goblet Squat		1-2	10-12
Chest Supported Row		1-2	8-10
Body Weight Split Squat		1-2	8-10
Push-ups		1-2	10-12
Loaded Carry	30-sec.	1-2	
Alternating Press		1-2	8-10

Week 2 / Day 1 – 3

Keep all exercises the same over the course of the first two weeks (6 exercise sessions). Change resistance accordingly and slow the cadence down for any or all body weight exercises you may be doing. If you are deconditioned you may need more recovery between each set of exercises. As fitness and work capacity improves, so too will the speed that you get through each session. If workouts end up taking longer than 30 minutes you will notice that your time over the coming weeks will most likely start to decrease. Wearing a heart rate monitor during both cardio and strength sessions will give you a better overall understanding of how your body is being challenged and how it handles the stress of exercise.

TBC30 Plan: Phase 1: Week 2 / Day 1

Exercise	Time	Sets	Reps
Warm-up			
Dynamic Warm-Up			
T-Pin or Foam Roller	5:00		
Mobility & Core			
Mobility work (4)	5:00		
Bird Dog		1-2	6-8
Prone Plank	45-sec.	1-2	
Glute Bridge		1-2	8-10
Side Plank	45-sec.	1-2	
Movement			
Med Ball or Goblet Squat		2	10-12
Chest Supported Row		2	8-10
Body Weight Split Squat		2	8-10
Push-ups		2	8-10
Loaded Carry	45-sec.	2	
Alternating Press		2	8-10

TBC30 Plan: Phase 1: Week 2 / Day 2

Exercise	Time	Sets	Reps
Warm-up			
Dynamic Warm-Up			
T-Pin or Foam Roller	5:00		
Mobility & Core			
Mobility work (4)	5:00		
Bird Dog		1-2	6-8
Prone Plank	45-sec.	1-2	
Glute Bridge		1-2	8-10
Side Plank	45-sec.	1-2	
Movement			
Med Ball or Goblet Squat		2	10-12
Chest Supported Row		2	8-10
Body Weight Split Squat		2	8-10
Push-ups		2	8-10
Loaded Carry	45-sec.	2	
Alternating Press		2	8-10

TBC30 Plan: Phase 1: Week 2 / Day 3

Exercise	Time	Sets	Reps
Warm-up			
Dynamic Warm-Up			
T-Pin or Foam Roller	5:00		
Mobility & Core			
Mobility work (4)	5:00		
Bird Dog		1-2	6-8
Prone Plank	45-sec.	1-2	
Glute Bridge		1-2	8-10
Side Plank	45-sec.	1-2	
Movement			
Med Ball or Goblet Squat		2	10-12
Chest Supported Row		2	8-10
Body Weight Split Squat		2	8-10
Push-ups		2	8-10
Loaded Carry	45-sec.	2	
Alternating Press		2	8-10

Week 3 / Day 1-3

There are a few changes on the exercise front for this week through week 4. For the Squat category you have a new exercise Barbell Back Squat. If you do not have access to an Olympic barbell simply substitute in a Dumbbell Squat. On the horizontal Pull category your new exercise for the next two weeks (6 sessions) is a one-arm dumbbell row. This can be performed off a bench or with both feet on the ground.

On the Lunge category you move from a Split Squat to a Reverse Lunge. For the horizontal push category your new exercise is a Bench Press, one of the better upper body multi-joint exercises: great for building overall strength. Stick with your loaded Carry – you could try switching whatever you were carrying during the first two weeks. For example, I recently moved from kettlebell Carries to Olympic (45-lbs.) plate Carries. Finally, your vertical Push category transitions from alternating Dumbbell Press to a Dumbbell Push Press. A great exercise using a small amount of hip extension to drive the dumbbells overhead. The idea is to stick to using the same exercises for 2-4 weeks before progressing to a newer, more challenge movement. Master the movement (movement competency) before loading up on the weight and moving to the next exercise too quickly.

TBC30 Plan: Phase 1: Week 3 / Day 1

Exercise	Time	Sets	Reps
Warm-up			
Dynamic Warm-Up			
T-Pin or Foam Roller	5:00		
Mobility & Core			
Mobility work (4)	5:00		
Bird Dog		1-2	6-8
Prone Plank	60-sec.	1-2	
Glute Bridge		1-2	8-10
Side Plank	60-sec.	1-2	
Movement			
Barbell Back Squat		2-3	10-12
One-Arm Row		2-3	8-10
Reverse Lunge		2-3	8-10
Bench Press		2-3	8-10
Loaded Carry	60-sec.	2-3	
Push Press		2-3	8-10

TBC30 Plan: Phase 1: Week 3 / Day 2

Exercise	Time	Sets	Reps
Warm-up			
Dynamic Warm-Up			
T-Pin or Foam Roller	5:00		
Mobility & Core			
Mobility work (4)	5:00		
Bird Dog		1-2	6-8
Prone Plank	60-sec.	1-2	
Glute Bridge		1-2	8-10
Side Plank	60-sec.	1-2	
Movement			
Barbell Back Squat		2-3	10-12
One-Arm Row		2-3	8-10
Reverse Lunge		2-3	8-10
Bench Press		2-3	8-10
Loaded Carry	60-sec.	2-3	
Push Press		2-3	8-10

TBC30 Plan: Phase 1: Week 3 / Day 3

Exercise	Time	Sets	Reps
Warm-up			
Dynamic Warm-Up			
T-Pin or Foam Roller	5:00		
Mobility & Core			
Mobility work (4)	5:00		
Bird Dog		1-2	6-8
Prone Plank	60-sec.	1-2	
Glute Bridge		1-2	8-10
Side Plank	60-sec.	1-2	
Movement			
Barbell Back Squat		2-3	10-12
One-Arm Row		2-3	8-10
Reverse Lunge		2-3	8-10
Bench Press		2-3	8-10
Loaded Carry	60-sec.	2-3	
Push Press		2-3	8-10

Week 4 / Day 1-3

This is your final week and the last three strength sessions in the program. Make them your best three training sessions. Stay with the same exercises used during week 3. During week 4 you move to three sets for exercises. If you're able to perform more than the suggested repetitions, increase your resistance by 10 percent or execute the movement using a slower cadence.

Following the completion of these three sessions you will need to complete your follow-up TBC30 assessment within the next day or two. Compare the differences from your baseline assessment.

TBC30 Plan: Phase 1: Week 4 / Day 1

Exercise	Time	Sets	Reps
Warm-up			
Dynamic Warm-Up			
T-Pin or Foam Roller	5:00		
Mobility & Core			
Mobility work (4)	5:00		
Bird Dog		1-2	6-8
Prone Plank	75-sec.	1-2	
Glute Bridge		1-2	8-10
Side Plank	30-sec.	1-2	
Movement			
Barbell Back Squat		3	10-12
One-Arm Row		3	8-10
Reverse Lunge		3	8-10
Bench Press		3	8-10
Loaded Carry	75-sec.	3	
Push Press		3	8-10

TBC30 Plan: Phase 1: Week 4 / Day 2

Exercise	Time	Sets	Reps
Warm-up			
Dynamic Warm-Up			
T-Pin or Foam Roller	5:00		
Mobility & Core			
Mobility work (4)	5:00		
Bird Dog		1-2	6-8
Prone Plank	75-sec.	1-2	
Glute Bridge		1-2	8-10
Side Plank	75-sec.	1-2	
Movement			
Barbell Back Squat		3	10-12
One-Arm Row		3	8-10
Reverse Lunge		3	8-10
Bench Press		3	8-10
Loaded Carry	75-sec.	3	
Push Press		3	8-10

TBC30 Plan: Phase 1: Week 4 / Day 3

Exercise	Time	Sets	Reps
Warm-up			
Dynamic Warm-Up			
T-Pin or Foam Roller	5:00		
Mobility & Core			
Mobility work (4)	5:00		
Bird Dog		1-2	6-8
Prone Plank	75-sec.	1-2	
Glute Bridge		1-2	8-10
Side Plank	75-sec.	1-2	
Movement			
Barbell Back Squat		3	10-12
One-Arm Row		3	8-10
Reverse Lunge		3	8-10
Bench Press		3	8-10
Loaded Carry	75-sec.	3	
Push Press		3	8-10

Final Thoughts on the Importance of Diet & Exercise

I hope this book has done a good job at presenting valid reasons, backed by science, on why nutrition and exercise are so important for improving your health and well being. The program will work for you if you follow and practice the TBC30 6 steps and become more mindful of what you're putting into your body to fuel it. But just in case it has not resonated with you yet, let me leave you with a few final statistics.

What Happens When You Don't Exercise?

As previously mentioned, more than a third of the U.S. population does not participate in any type of exercise.

When you do not exercise your body will change in profound ways. One of the first things you notice when exercise is non-existent is potential weight gain. Research shows when you gain weight, you have an increased risk for high blood pressure, heart disease and type 2 diabetes. Being overweight makes both exercise and activities of daily living harder because additional stress is placed on your joints when you walk, run or jog.

There are also many changes that take place inside your body when you don't exercise regularly. Bones begin to lose density with age and limited or no weight-bearing exercise plays a major role in osteoporosis, or brittle bones. Your body responds to the demands you put on it, and if you do not exercise, your connective tissue, muscles and bones weaken over time.

Lack of exercise can also lead to a diminished sense of well being. Your body loses muscle strength and tone and your self-esteem can suffer as a result. Aerobic exercises like swimming, biking or running stimulates your body to release endorphins, a neurotransmitter that plays a big role in the function of the central nervous system.

There are at least twenty different types of endorphins and some people think these are responsible for enabling that well-known "runners high" you can get during exercise. Researchers, however, often believe that the endocannabinoid system may be more responsible for that feeling.

Finally, a lack of exercise has been associated with the following: a loss of muscle size and strength, aerobic capacity, a decrease in mitochondria (powerhouse of the cell), changes in mood, and a decrease in energy level and don't let me forget sex drive.

Once you have completed your program you will need to complete your follow-up assessment. This includes the same group of tests that you used initially for your baseline testing. Best of luck and remember that you now have a "Game Plan" to follow, so work the plan and trust the process. Remember, when difficulty arises, fall back on the TBC30 strategies you've learned and remember my favorite quote from Henry Ford:

"Whether you think you can or think you can't, you're right."

Please email me at woodspg@gmail.com and let me know how you made out after you completed your program. Let us also know if you're interested in our web-based coaching services at michaelwoodfitness.com – Stay Strong!

Resources

Scientific Research Publications

Basso, J. C. & Suzuki, W. A. (2017). The effects of acute exercise on mood, cognition, neurophysiology, and neurochemical pathways: a review. *Brain Plasticity*, 2(2): 127.

Basu, S., Yoffe, P., Hills, N., Lustig, R. H. (2013). The relationship of sugar to population-level diabetes prevalence: an econometric analysis of repeated cross-sectional data. *PLOS ONE* 8(2), e57873.

Bohannon R. W., Peolsson A., et al. (2006). Reference values for adult grip strength measured with a Jamar dynamometer: a descriptive meta-analysis, *Physiotherapy*, 92(1): 11-15.

Boschmann, M., Steiniger, J., Hille, U., Tank, J., Adams, F., Sharma, A. M., Klaus, S., Luft, F. C., Jordan, J. (2003). Water-induced thermogenesis. *The Journal of Clinical Endocrinology and Metabolism*, 88(12), 6015-6019.

Burstein, R., Epstein, Y. et. al. (1990). Effect of an acute bout of exercise on glucose disposal in human obesity. *Journal Applied Physiology*, 69(1): 299-304.

Coughlin, S. & Stewart, J. (2016). Use of consumer wearable devices to promote physical activity: a review of health intervention studies. *Journal Environmental Health Science*, 2(6): doi:10.15436/2378-6841.16.1123

Doherty, T. J. (2001). The influence of aging and sex on skeletal muscle mass and strength. *Current Opinions Clinical Nutrition Metabolic Care*, (4), 503-508.

Flegal, K. M., Carroll, M. D., Kit, B. K., Ogden, C. L. (2012). Prevalence of obesity and trends in the distribution of body mass index among US adults, 1999–2010. *Journal of American Medical Association*, 307(5), 491–7.

Fujioka, K., Greenway, F. et. al. (2006). The effects of grapefruit on weight and insulin resistance: relationship to the metabolic syndrome. *Journal Medicinal Food*, 9(1): 49-54.

Gale, S. M., Castracane, V. D., and Mantzoros, C. S., (2004). Energy homeostasis, obesity and eating disorders: recent advances in endocrinology. *Journal of Nutrition*, 134(2), 295–298.

Gardner, C. D. et. al., (2018). Effect of low-fat vs low-carbohydrate diet on 12-month weight loss in overweight adults and the association with genotype pattern or insulin secretion. *Journal American Medical Association*, 319(7): 667-679. doi:10.1001/jama.2018.0245

Gillen, J. B., Martin, B. J., et. al. (2016). Twelve weeks of sprint interval training improves indices of cardiometabolic health similar to traditional endurance training despite a five-fold lower exercise volume and time commitment. *PLOS ONE*, doi:10.1371/journal.pone.0154075

Hartman, S. J. et. al. (2018). Patterns of fitbit use and activity levels throughout a physical activity intervention: exploratory analysis from a randomized controlled trial. *JMIR Mhealth Uhealth*, 6(2), e29.

Krogh-Madsen R, Thyfault J. P, Broholm C, Mortensen O. H., Olsen R. H., Mounier R., Plomgaard P., van Hall G., Booth F. W., and Pedersen, B. K. (2010). A 2-wk reduction of ambulatory activity attenuates peripheral insulin sensitivity. *J Appl Physiology*, 108(5):1034-1040.

Leong, D. P, Teo K. K. et. al., (2015). Prognostic value of grip strength: findings from the prospective urban rural epidemiology (PURE) study. *Lancet*, 386(9990): 266-273. doi:10.1016/S0140-6736(14)62000-6

Meredith, C. N., Zackin, M. J., Frontera, W. R., Evans, W. J. (1989). Dietary protein requirements and body protein metabolism in endurance-trained men. *Journal Applied Physiology*, 66(6): 2850-2856.

Morenga, L. T., Mallard, S., Mann, J. (2013). Dietary sugars and body weight: systematic review and meta-analyses of randomized controlled trials and cohort studies. *British Medical Journal*, 346. doi:10.1136/bmj.e7492

Mozaffarian, D., Hao, T., Rimm, E. B., Willett, W. C., and Hu, F. B., (2011). Changes in diet and lifestyle and long-term weight gain in women and men. *New England Journal Medicine*, (364), 2392-2404.

Nanda, B., Balde, J. et al. (2013). The acute effects of a single bout of moderate-intensity aerobic exercise on cognitive functions in healthy adult males. *Journal Clinical Diagnostic Research* 7(9): 1883–1885.

Nedeltcheva, A. V., et al., (2010). Insufficient Sleep Undermines Dietary Efforts to Reduce Adiposity. *Annals Internal Medicine*, (153), 435-441.

Popkin, B. M., et al., (2006). A new proposed guidance system for beverage consumption in the united states. *Journal Clinical Nutrition*, (83), 529-542.

Popkin, B. M., Armstrong, L. E., et al., (2006). A new proposed guidance system for beverage consumption in the United States. *The American Journal of Clinical Nutrition*, 83(3): 529–542.

Pollock, N. K., Bundy, V., Kanto, W., Davis, C. L., Bernard, P. J., et al., (2011). Greater fructose consumption is associated with cardiometabolic risk markers and visceral adiposity in adolescents. *Journal of Nutrition*, 142(2), 251. doi:10.3945/jn.111.150219

Poon, L. W., Clayton, G., Martin, P., et al. (1989). Individual similarities and differences of the oldest-old in the georgia centenarian study. *The Gerontologist*, (29), 43.

Rabin C, & Bock B. (2011). Desired features of smartphone applications' promoting physical activity. *Telemed J E Health*, 17(10):801-803

Roxburgh, B. H., et al. (2014). Is moderate intensity exercise training combined with high intensity interval training more effective at improving cardiorespiratory fitness than moderate intensity exercise training alone? *Journal Sports Science Medicine*, 13(3): 702-707.

Samani, A. & Heath, M. (2018). Executive related oculomotor control is improved following a 10-min single-bout of aerobic exercise: evidence from the antisaccade task. *Neuropsychologia*, doi:10.1016/j.neuropsychologia.2017.11.02

Schneider; et al., (2010). The predictive value of different measures of obesity for incident cardiovascular events and mortality. *The Journal of Clinical Endocrinology & Metabolism*, 95(4): 1777–1785.

Schulze, B. M, Manson, J. E., Ludwig, D. S. et al., (2004). Sugar-sweetened beverages, weight gain, and incidence of type 2 diabetes in young and middle-aged women. *Journal American Medical Association*, 292(8): 927-934. doi:10.1001/jama.292.8.927

Stanhope, K. L., Bremer, A. A., Medici, V., Nakajima, K., Ito, Y., Nakano, T., Chen, G., et al. (2011). Consumption of fructose and high fructose corn syrup increase postprandial triglycerides, ldl-cholesterol, and apolipoprotein-b in young men and women. *Journal of Clinical Endocrinology and Metabolism*, 96(10), doi:10.1210/jc.2011-1251

Spiegel, K., et. al., (2004). Sleep curtailment in healthy young men is associated with decreased leptin levels, elevated ghrelin levels, and increased hunger and appetite. *Annals of Internal Medicine*, 141(11), 846-85.
Thijssen, D. J., Redington, A., George, K. P. (2018). Association of exercise preconditioning with immediate cardioprotection. *Journal American Medical Association Cardiology*, 3(2): 169-176. doi:10:1001/jamacardio.2017.4495

Tudor-Locke C, Ainsworth B. E., Whitt M. C., et al. (2001). The relationship between pedometer-determined ambulatory activity and body composition variables. *Int. J Obesity*, 25: 1571-1578.

Tudor-Locke C, Bassett D. R. Jr. (2004). How many steps/day are enough? Preliminary pedometer indices for public health. *Sports Med.*, 34(1):1-8

Tudor-Locke C, Ham S. A., et al. Descriptive epidemiology of pedometer-determined physical activity. *Med Sci Sports Exerc.*, 36(9): 1567-1573

Tudor-Locke C, Schuna J. M. (2012). Steps to preventing Type 2 diabetes: exercise, walk more, or sit less? *Front Endocrinol.*, 3:142

White, P. L., et al. (1955). Nutritive values of crops, nutrient content and protein quality of quinua and cañihua, edible seed products of the andes mountains. *Journal Agricultural Food Chemistry*, 3(6): 531-534.

Wilmot, E. G., & Edwardson, C. L. (2012). Sedentary time in adults and the association with diabetes, cardiovascular disease and death: systematic review and meta-analysis, *Diabetologia*, 55(11), 2895-905. doi:10.1007/s00125-012-2677-z

Books

Dweck, C. (2016). *Mindset: The new psychology of success.* New York, NY: Ballantine.

Evans, W., & Rosenberg, I. (1992). *Biomarkers.* New York, NY: Simon and Schuster.

Harlan, T. (2011). *Just tell me what to eat.* Cambridge, MA: Da Capo Press.

Harris, D. (2017). *Meditation for fidgety skeptics.* New York, NY: Spiegel & Grau.

Hutchinson A. (2018). *Endure: Mind, body, and the curiously elastic limits of human performance.* New York, NY: William Morrow.

Kesteller, J. (2015). *The joy of half a cookie.* New York, NY: Perigee Book.

Rogers, M. A., & Evans, W. J. (1993). Changes in skeletal muscle with aging: effects of exercise training. *Exercise and Sport Science Reviews.* Baltimore, MD: Williams and Wilkins.

Taubes, G. (2007). *Good calories, bad calories.* New York, NY: Alfred Knopf.

Witkin, B. R., & Altschuld, J. W. (1995). *Planning and conducting needs assessments: A practical guide.* Thousand Oaks, CA: Sage Publications.

Web-based Articles & Publications

Bernado, R. (2017, November). 2016's Fattest States in America. Wallet Hub

Centers for Disease Control, Division of Nutrition, Physical Activity, and Obesity, National Center for Chronic Disease Prevention and Health Promotion.

Centers for Disease and Control and Morbidity and Mortality (1999).

Hanh, T.N. (2010, August). Five Steps to Mindfulness. Mindful Magazine.

Jameson, M. (2010, December). A Reversal on Carbs. Los Angeles Times.

Taubes, G. (2011, April). Is Sugar Toxic? New York Times.

National Sleep Foundation, Sleep in America Poll (2003). National Sleep Foundation, Washington, DC.

Martinez, R. (2015). Prevalence of Overweight and Obesity Visualization. Health Intelligence. World Health Data Charts, 2014.

National Center for Health Statistics (2005). Quick stats: percentage of adults who reported an average of 66 h of sleep per 24-h period, by sex and age group United States, 1985 and 2004. Morbidity and Mortality Weekly Report.

Webb, W. B., Agnew, H.W. (1975, July). Are we chronically sleep deprived? Bulletin of the Psychonomic Society, 6(1), 47–48.

World Health Organization (1999). Definition, diagnosis, and classification of diabetes mellitus and its complications: report of a WHO consultation. Part I: diagnosis and classification of diabetes mellitus.

Helpful Links & Apps

PWC. (2016, May). The Wearable Life 2.0: connected living in a wearable world.
http://www.pwc.com/us/en/industry/entertainment-media/assets/pwc-cis-wearables.pdf

Myfitnesspal app - http://myfitnesspal.com

Welltory app – http://welltory.com

FitBit app – http://fitbit.com

Headspace app – http://headspace.com

T-Pin Vector – http://tpinmuscletherapy.com/

Ascent protein – http://ascentprotein.com

ElliptiGo – http://www.elliptigo.com

Inside Tracker -http://insidetracker.com

About the Author

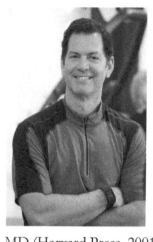

Michael Wood, CSCS, is a certified strength & conditioning specialist and nutrition coach (PN1). He is a nationally recognized fitness expert and author of *The TBC30 plan: A 6-Step Diet & Exercise Strategy for Life* (Amazon Digital, 2017). His exercise programs have appeared in two other books, *The 30-Minute Fitness Solution* by JoAnn Manson, MD (Harvard Press, 2001) and *Cut Your Cholesterol* by David Katz, MD (Reader's Digest, 2003). Michael is the co-author of ten scientific research papers and abstracts as a result of exercise research completed at the USDA Human Nutrition Research Center on Aging at Tufts University in Boston. He has been featured in media and print publications such as *U.S. News & World Report, Boston Magazine, Men's Health, Prevention, Best Life, Men's Fitness, Boston Globe, Denver Post* and *Delta Sky Magazine*. His exercise programs are completed more than 200,000 times each month by members at Koko FitClub franchises across the U.S. and Canada. Michael was a former assistant strength & conditioning coach at UConn where he also attended graduate school. Michael was named twice by *Men's Journal* as one of the "Top 100 Trainers in America" and voted Best of Boston by *Boston Magazine*. He lives in Massachusetts on Cape Cod with his wife and daughter. Michael's coaching services and products are available.

To inquire, please visit: www.MichaelWoodFitness.com